Y0-BVF-035

YOGINI:
Ageless Women, Timeless Tradition

Patricia Gottlieb Shapiro

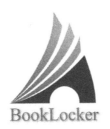

BookLocker

Copyright © 2019 Patricia Gottlieb Shapiro, MSW, RYT

ISBN: 978-1-64438-788-7

All rights reserved. No part of this publication may be reproduced, stored in a retrieval system, or transmitted in any form or by any means, electronic, mechanical, recording or otherwise, without the prior written permission of the author.

Published by BookLocker.com, Inc., St. Petersburg, Florida.

Printed on acid-free paper.

BookLocker.com, Inc.
2019

First Edition

Also by Patricia Gottlieb Shapiro

- *The Privilege of Aging: Portraits of Twelve Jewish Women*
- *Coming Home to Yourself: Eighteen Wise Women Reflect on Their Journeys*
- *Yoga for Women at Midlife & Beyond: A Home Companion*
- *Always My Child: A Parent's Guide to Understanding Your Gay, Lesbian, Bisexual, Transgendered or Questioning Son or Daughter* (with coauthor)
- *Heart to Heart: Deepening Women's Friendships at Midlife*
- *My Turn: Women's Search for Self After the Children Leave*
- *A Parent's Guide to Childhood and Adolescent Depression*
- *Women, Mentors and Success* (with coauthor)
- *Caring for the Mentally Ill*

For Dick

Contents

Introduction

Doing yoga as an older woman can transform how you feel about yourself and how you view aging. Listen to what Rayna Griffin had to say: "Yoga really changed me. It helped me open my heart and mind, and expand as a person. I'm digging deeper now. I'm learning, growing and discovering more about myself every day." She is 69, an age at which psychologists in the past thought people stopped growing.

Sadly, many older people do stop growing. They still spend their "golden" years in a static way: sitting on the porch constantly checking their email or watching cable television all day. But for those who do want to keep developing, the later years can be rich and rewarding.

We now know that growth does not stop at age 65. The years beyond 65 are their own developmental period, just like midlife and adolescence: a stage of *becoming,* not just being. The psychologist Erik Erikson told us that after age 65 you have a choice between integrity and despair. If you choose integrity, the later years can be a period of expanding mentally, strengthening physically, deepening emotionally, and evolving spiritually.

That's the positive side of aging. But, of course, everything is not all rosy as we age; another side exists as well. It is also a period of tremendous loss. We face losses in relation to our own health and wellbeing, we lose friends and partners to illness and death, and ultimately, we face our own mortality.

We know we're not perfect and hope we're not finished growing, but we're in a very different space than when we were younger. We are not constantly second guessing ourselves or desperately seeking approval of everyone we meet. If "they" don't like us, that's their problem. We're fine with who we are. And if our "fine" is a little shaky, yoga can give us the confidence we need.

Jean Backlund, 82, whom you'll meet in these pages, noticed a big change in her attitude after she had taken yoga classes for a while. "When I was younger, I was always somewhat quiet and introverted," she told me. "But now I can stand up in front of a group and talk. I use my relaxed breathing techniques before I speak to a group and I'm fine, much to my amazement."

The media tells us that 70 is the new 50, and there's actually some truth to this. Seventy is no longer old, but it's also very different from 50 and 60. Like the fifties, the sixties and seventies can be full of vitality and life, but the later years contain a sober twist: there's a recognition of how fleeting time is and how precious each moment. We have seen our lives and our friends' lives transformed on a dime with a shocking diagnosis of ovarian cancer, a heart attack on a treadmill, or a brutal car accident—reminding us that each day is indeed a gift. And on those days when "nothing" happens and life seems quiet and boring, we remember these days are precious, too, as this familiar quote from author Mary Jean Orion reminds us: "Normal day, let me be aware of the treasure you are."

Many have said, in fact, that this is the best time in their lives, that they've never been more content, and that their days are richer and fuller than in the past. Maybe the reason for this richness is that we know—whether we talk about it or not—that our days are finite, and thus, more cherished.

These are the issues that form the background of this book, **YOGINI: *Ageless Women, Timeless Tradition.*** It contains the stories of ten women—narratives of physical and emotional healing, of overcoming adversity, and of spiritual renewal. These women come from all parts of the United States, study in different yoga traditions, and range in age from 63 to 85.

Some women are trying yoga for the first time at age 65 or 70; others have come back to yoga at that age after a hiatus of 20 or 30 years. Still others, like Ana Franklin, have been practicing consistently for 50 years. What keeps her practicing after all these years? "I could have gone off the deep end if I didn't have my practice," she said. "My practice kept me sane and alive."

In this book, you'll meet women who only go to class once a week but have incorporated the principles of yoga into their lives. That makes them a serious yoga student to me. Women like this are living their yoga, what's known as "off the mat," even though they may only be "on the mat" (practicing in class or at home) once a week. What counts is how important yoga is to them, how passionate they feel about it, and how pervasive its principles are to their actions and behaviors.

I interviewed many women to find the ten who appear in this book. Part of the inspiration for this book was an interview with Alice Ladas, age 96. Alice said yoga was her "constant companion," that she mostly did yoga to remain healthy and flexible. She would certainly win the prize for doing yoga the longest. She started in the 1940s doing yoga with Jack LaLanne and followed along as she watched Lilias Folan's television program, "Yoga and You," as she raised her two young daughters.

In other situations you'll read about, yoga does its magic in unknown ways. Take painter and sculptor Rayna Griffin: she had lost all inspiration until she discovered yoga, which freed and inspired her in new ways. Or Jean Backlund, who refused to leave her house for a year after her husband died. When her neighbors dragged Jean to a yoga class, it turned her life around.

What's different about these stories is that the women are all beyond midlife. They are practicing regularly at an age when conventional wisdom says they are too old for yoga, yet they are reaping its many benefits. Strength, flexibility, and balance are more available, as well as the calm and peace of mind so important as we get older and face the many challenges that accompany aging.

CONNECTION AND CAMRADERIE

When older women practice together, something different happens. So many women have told me how incompetent they feel when they're in a yoga class with twentysomethings and the younger women are standing on their heads or contorting themselves into positions impossible for older bodies.

Lillian Weilerstein, 83, whom you'll meet in these pages, told me, "I never did a handstand. You make your choices. You don't worry about what someone else is doing. When I was younger, I was more self-conscious. After I turned 80, I didn't care what everyone thinks."

When older women practice with their peers, they feel a sense of camaraderie and community. A bond is created when they breathe together and move together. There's a degree of comfort because they know that these women are like them. Everyone has "something" going on. Whether it's a bad back, osteoporosis, or cancer, everyone knows that the others in class have their own unique challenges and their own source of *duhkha* (suffering).

For some older women, *duhkha* stems from physical or health challenges like the ones just mentioned. For others, it is emotional difficulties that create *duhkha*. They include making decisions about how and where to live, coming to terms with regrets, contending with issues and anxieties about getting older, and losing friends and family members.

Whether our own personal *duhkha* comes from physical or emotional pain, we can learn from it. Among the things we learn from our own suffering and by studying ourselves through yoga are patience, compassion, and gratitude.

And we gain wisdom. Although we may not sense it every day, our long lives have indeed granted us wisdom. When my daughter calls and says, "Mom, I need some motherly advice" or a friend says, "I need to talk to you," I know that I have learned a few things in my 70+ years, and what I can offer in terms of compassion, empathy and understanding is hard won.

YOGA FOR OLDER WOMEN

Time goes faster as we age. The only way to slow it down is to live in the moment and appreciate that moment. For that, yoga is our guide. If we can learn to breathe and focus on a single breath in class, we can take that skill off the mat and make it part of our everyday life.

Of course, you can do yoga at any age, but something different happens when you practice as an older woman. You have a seasoned perspective that you didn't have when you were younger. You have a long history and by now, you know what's important and what's not. You know your body well and know how to listen to it and heed what you hear.

Your goals are different as you age and you have more compassionate for yourself. You're not striving for a perfect pose as you did when you were younger. Instead, you want to protect and preserve your physical and emotional health. That means if you wake up particularly stiff one morning, you may need to do more warm-ups than usual. Or if you're feeling sluggish or tired, you may choose to practice in a chair. There's nothing wrong with this: It's where you are at this particular moment on this particular day, and this, too, will change.

As you age, function becomes more important than form as it becomes more and more challenging to recreate that ideal classical pose. Your body just won't do certain things anymore; it won't move in certain ways. On the positive side, this gives you an opportunity to learn about yourself *while you are in the posture.* You do the pose from the inside out. As you practice, you ask yourself: How does this feel on the inside? How is my body responding? You observe yourself as you practice *(svadyaya)* and make modifications as needed.

What's more, you begin to realize that the purpose of yoga is not to master a posture. It's about *using a posture to understand and transform yourself.* Postures are your tools to do that. So, if you come to class remembering that this is not about a posture, but about you and use a posture to understand how you feel and how you function, then you truly grasp the meaning of yoga.

Of course, you want to be strong and flexible—that's one of the reasons you practice, but as you get older, you want to go deeper. You want to dive beneath the surface to reflect on some of the principles that make yoga so universal and so timeless. Through studying and reflecting on these concepts, you get to know yourself in a deeper, more fundamental and spiritual way.

I've been teaching yoga to women at midlife and older since 1999. I'm open to teaching men but they haven't come to my classes, so over the years, I've shifted my attention to solely focus on women.

At the end of each of my classes, I share some of the ideas from the *Yoga Sutra* with my students and show how they are relevant to their lives today. These concepts then become the focus of the meditation that follows. We've covered the *yamas* (our attitudes toward others), the *niyamas* (our attitudes toward ourselves), *duhkha* (emotional suffering), *avidya* (incorrect knowledge, false understanding and clouded perceptions), and many other concepts.

Tracey Fox, a 76-year-old woman who has been studying with me for about a year, spoke for many of my students when she told me recently, "You probably see me tear up during the meditation. It always brings up something for me, either during class or later in the day." This is just one example of the subtlety and unexpected effects of yoga practice.

MY YOGA CONNECTION

The first time I did yoga I was in my early 50s. I was going through a difficult time and desperately needed something to help me cope. Everyone was talking about yoga so I decided to give it a try. I loved it from the moment I walked into my first class in a small studio in a rehabbed section of Philadelphia. Everything was completely white: the walls, flooring, pillows. Even before I started moving and breathing consciously, I felt a huge sense of relief. I had walked in uptight and edgy, not having slept the night before. When I walked out after that first class, I was in a very different place. I knew the problems were still there but somehow, they seemed more distant. Yes, they were still serious, but I had developed a calm that enabled me to handle them better. I was able to be more thoughtful in my responses and less reactive.

From the nurturing I received and the connection I felt, I couldn't wait to go back for more classes. There was no question in my mind that yoga would be an important piece of my life from then on.

Since that first class over twenty years ago, yoga has been my daily companion. In my 2006 book, *Yoga for Women at Midlife & Beyond: A Home Companion,* I wrote: "Yoga is a homecoming: a coming home to ourselves." And that's exactly how I feel—every single day.

My yoga practice sustains me: it keeps me steady and grounded. But it's more than that too: Yoga has been my salvation when challenges arise and I need to handle *duhkha.*

A few years ago, when I was experiencing writer's block, yoga helped me return to my other "home," writing. After completing my last book, I didn't think I'd write another one. With no inspiration, my ideas had dried up and I felt that my life as a writer was over. Nonetheless, I continued to call myself a writer— even though I wasn't writing. During this period, I knew something was missing. I felt unsettled and unproductive, but I couldn't quite figure out what was going on. I took poetry classes, dabbled in book arts, and sampled the rich cultural scene in Santa

Fe, New Mexico. Although these activities were enjoyable, they didn't satisfy me on a visceral level as writing does.

Yoga was the one thing that supported me during this disconcerting period. Through doing meditation, yoga and breath work, I was able to connect to who I truly am, reflect on what I wanted to do with the rest of my life, and gain some clarity about what mattered most to me. It was through this process that I discovered a focus for my next book. I was home!

It doesn't matter whether I'm standing on one foot in Tree Pose on a mat in my own bedroom in Santa Fe or in a hotel room in St. Petersburg, Russia: Yoga transports me to a place without boundaries, a place of inner peace and calm where I feel centered and grounded. When I come off the mat, I take that feeling with me and it gives me comfort and confidence to be myself— wherever I am and whomever I'm with.

BECOMING A TEACHER

For seven or eight years, I attended class regularly and continued to love doing yoga. I always felt relaxed and clear after I left, but I had no desire to practice at home or delve any deeper into the study or philosophy of yoga. I decided to become a teacher so I could share my passion with others. A personal practice is critical in becoming a teacher, I learned on the very first day. It furthers her own growth and development.

That was all the motivation I needed. I started practicing at home every morning. Once I started, I had no problem keeping it up. I'd wash my face, brush my teeth, and throw out my mat: my morning ritual. I loved the stretching and deep breathing when I was half awake. I liked the way I felt after doing my practice—calm, centered and focused—ready to start my day. If I skipped a day, I noticed I was more reactive to people and situations that arose during the day.

The week after I finished my teacher training, a long-time teacher left the studio and I was asked to take over her class for older women. That was 1999. Two years later, we moved to Santa Fe. It took a few years to get my teaching off the ground. Initially, I taught in different venues and students came and went. But over time, I developed a core group of committed students who signed up for series after series.

YOGA AND PD

In the fall of 2016 I was diagnosed with Parkinson's Disease (PD). About six months before my diagnosis, I noticed some subtle changes. I had a tremor in my right hand that I never had before. My handwriting changed. It kept getting smaller and smaller until it was hardly legible. And I was very stiff when I woke up in the morning.

When I saw my internist, she wasn't that concerned. Even if it were PD, she said, my symptoms were so mild and it was so early that I wouldn't need medication. I decided I'd just put it out of my mind and move on with my life. Easier said than done.

Much as I'd like to report otherwise, at this point, my practice did not serve me well. The elephant in the room was just too large. Where I was usually calm and focused when I practiced, I was now agitated and scattered. I was going through the poses mechanically. My mind was all over the place. If it were PD, what would that mean for my life? What would have to change? Could I still teach? What about driving? Then, I'd switch gears—It can't be PD. It must be an essential tremor, like a friend has had for 45 years.

Then, what symptoms would I get and how would they progress? Of course, I read about Michael J. Fox, but I only knew two people personally with PD. Both had dealt with the disease for about ten years. One, in her early 80s, had no visible symptoms; the other, a few years younger, used a walker. Where would I fall in this spectrum? Please God, I bargained, just give me ten good years so I can see my four grandchildren go off to college.

I decided I needed a diagnosis to calm me down. Then I would know what I was dealing with and could focus my energy on finding treatments I was comfortable considering. When a neurologist confirmed my diagnosis, it was still a shock although I wasn't really surprised because, as I said earlier, I was having symptoms for about six months before I was diagnosed.

But Parkinson's Disease? No one in my family had Parkinson's. Cancer, yes. Heart disease, of course. Part of me wondered, is this a mistake? But deep down, I knew it was the correct diagnosis.

From that point on, I was calm and focused as I researched the disease, explored different treatment methods, and looked for the most natural ways to treat it. My yoga practice became (and still is) an essential part of my treatment. Every morning I go in my study, throw out my yoga mat and stand, facing the rising sun, hands in prayer position, and recite the following *bhavana* (intention):

Let the healing powers of the sun wash over me and heal me, circling my heart, moving down my arms to my fingertips, down through my trunk, my legs, grounding me to the earth, and enveloping me with healing. Let these powers slow the progression of the disease, quiet my tremor, soften the stiffness and keep me healthy.

I then do my practice, which includes *asana, pranayama,* chanting and a short meditation—a calming foundation for starting my day, bringing me home to myself.

WHY THIS BOOK NOW?

When my previous book, The *Privilege of Aging*, came out in August 2013, I announced that this was my last book. Friends and family laughed at me because they had heard this comment before. They knew I'd write another book. But I felt differently this time: I had written nine books and that was enough. I didn't want to deal with the pressure and intensity of writing another book. I wanted to enjoy myself more and work less. After all, I was about to turn 70.

The first year after I finished *The Privilege of Aging*, I was busy traveling and promoting it. I didn't think about writing. But as the one-year mark rolled around, I started to miss writing. When I heard people talk of their creative projects, I felt envious. I wanted to create something, too. I felt like something was missing from my life, but I didn't have an idea for a book. I decided to write a memoir for my children and grandchildren. I fleshed out an outline, wrote some essays, and developed a structure. Within a year, I had completed that project. It was gratifying that my children were so appreciative and that I had created a beautiful legacy for them and my grandchildren, but it didn't satisfy me in the same way that writing a "real" book does.

I then took on the editorship of *Legacy*, the quarterly newsletter of the New Mexico Jewish Historical Society. It was challenging on many levels and very satisfying, but I wasn't writing. As I inched toward two years as editor, I realized that something was still missing. And that "something" was writing.

Then three things happened within a month—all related to my teaching yoga. I received an email from a former student of mine who had moved to Washington state thanking me for the "gift" of yoga that I had given her when she was contemplating hip surgery. Just what was that gift?

Next, I learned that one of my current students was formerly homeless. She now has an apartment, lives on a shoestring, and has become an advocate for the homeless. What's her story and how has yoga helped her?

Lastly, a woman called after receiving my name from a former student and told me that she wants to get back into yoga but she has fibromyalgia and arthritis, among other medical problems, and she wasn't sure she was strong enough to handle the class. We had a long talk and I invited her to try a class and see if she liked it. If she didn't, she didn't have to take the series. She came to class the next day and seemed to participate comfortably. After class I asked her how it was for her. A big smile spread across her face as she said, "I feel like I've come home."

Even with the scant information I had about these three women, a light went off in my head and I knew I had an idea for book #10. Their experiences told me that there must be many more stories around that show how yoga has touched older women's lives and transformed them.

THE OLDER YOGINIS FEATURED

This book contains ten women's stories—eight individuals and a friendship that joins two women in a love of yoga. They are stories of physical and emotional healing, of adversity overcome, and of spiritual renewal. In each chapter, you'll get to know an older woman as a yogini. You'll hear her speak in her own words about how yoga has impacted on her life and how she has evolved as a result of yoga being a part of her later years. At the beginning of each chapter, her photograph in a favorite yoga pose will let you visualize her as you read. Below her photo, a quote from one of her interviews captures an important point.

Including each woman's photo was deliberate, because many older women feel invisible—their presence ignored and their words disregarded. By giving them their own chapter and photo, I hope to send a message that these women do matter. The form of their yoga pose may not be perfect, but they are doing their best. The fact that they're doing yoga in later life needs to be recognized.

You never see an older woman on the cover of *Yoga Journal*. Women on the covers are young, slim and attractive. As baby boomers age, they will identify less with the women on these covers and be searching for role models who look more like them. The women in this book, none household names, can inspire and hearten.

In their own words, these ten women will tell you what makes yoga so compelling, so necessary and so gratifying as they get older. If you're not a yogini yet and you're over 60, I hope they will inspire you to try yoga, no matter what your age, your body size or shape, or your health issues. If you're already practicing yoga, reading other women's stories and struggles will encourage you to continue on this path. This is an opportunity to open your mind, body and spirit to the wonders of yoga. Let it guide you and support you in the years ahead.

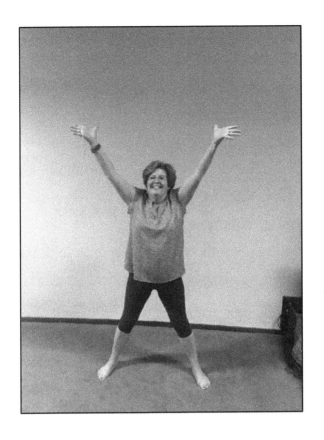

"My purpose is to express joy through my art and my life."

--Rayna Griffin

Rayna Griffin, 69: Gaining Inspiration

When Rayna Griffin attended her first yoga class at age 65, she knew she had come home. "It was so magical, I felt like crying," she told me. "It was just what I needed for my life and my head."

Truth be told, she had attended one other yoga class—a Hot Yoga class—15 years earlier. She didn't realize that "hot" referred to the temperature of the room and that the thermostat was purposely set high. Rayna thought it meant the "in" thing to do. Dripping with perspiration and getting more and more uncomfortable by the minute, she finally burst out loud: "Why doesn't someone turn on the A.C?" The room was silent. That experience convinced Rayna that yoga was not for her. She didn't take another class until she met her present yoga teacher, Naomi Rose (see Chapter 3 for Naomi's story), at the post office in Sedona, Arizona two years ago. She invited Rayna to try a class.

The old adage, "When the student is ready, the teacher will appear," certainly applied to Rayna. She was ripe for the effects of yoga. "I was dead inside for six years. I was spiraling down into a depression. I had a lot of worries about finances. My husband's profession came to a halt," she told me.

"I had done art my whole life but when life got crazy, nothing came to me," she said. "I just sat there. I shut down. I went on Prozac but I still couldn't do anything creative. Prozac stopped me from feeling like I wanted to cry all the time, even though I had a good life, a solid marriage, and a wonderful family. It somehow took away the feeling of aloneness and being lost, but I couldn't find joy and peace in myself. Before Prozac, I wondered why I was even on this planet and what I had to offer. Over my lifetime, I had done painting, sculpting, water colors, all kinds of art. For six years, nothing."

Art is just one of the things that Rayna pursued in her unconventional life. In 1972 as newlyweds, she and her husband John moved to Nairobi, Kenya, and opened a "hippie craft store." They sold pottery, leather goods, candles, clothing and local jewelry. She ran the shop while John ran the workshop that trained and employed six local Kenyans. They stayed there for six and a half years.

When they left Kenya in 1978, Rayna and John bought an RV and traveled the western states for six months with their two sons, ages one and three. In the course of their travels, they fell in love with Sedona, Arizona, and bought a house within a day. Rayna was a stay-at-home mom while the boys were young, throwing herself into community service. Among other activities, she was a Boy Scout troop leader, she started a recycling program in town, she was on a number of boards, and she taught art in several different local schools. Throughout these years, she always made art in some form and often sold her watercolors in local galleries.

The recession hit them hard in 2009 and 2010: her husband's custom home business came to a halt when the building industry in Sedona dried up. They lost a considerable amount of money in lots they owned to build homes on. They decided they needed to do something else for income. They heard from a friend that olive oil shops were a good investment with the growing trend in healthy eating. So, they opened a shop in Scottsdale, Arizona.

"I'm a small-town country girl. The only time we would go to the big city (Phoenix) was to go to the airport and fly somewhere," she told me. "I had to say goodbye to several art-related boards that I was on, try to get my head around owning and running a retail shop two-plus hours away from home, and dealing with big-city life."

They traveled each week the two and a half hours back and forth to the shop and worked three full days. She had to learn to operate a complicated cash register, integrate bookkeeping and inventory systems, and handle all personnel issues—while mastering the culture of olive oils from around the world.

"Long hours and a challenging new life for me at age 60, and both of us learning by the seat of our pants—wow! My brain was always exhausted and filled with business ideas or problems. My only creative outlet was decorating the shop for the seasons and making signs. I needed that artistic expression so badly!" she said.

"When I came back to Sedona after three days in Phoenix, I had no inspiration or energy for painting or being creative. Zero!! No time for art. My studio sat waiting for me, but I had no motivation, and nothing to express in art. I felt like a big part of me was gone. My mind and body were always racing to catch up with housework, laundry, bills, and groceries. Then organizing items needed or placing orders for the shop.

"I felt sooo divided as a person: part of me here and part of me in retail mode. My stomach was always in a flutter and my heart and mind felt like they were always racing. And I was living with a husband who had to leave a 30-year construction career and learn retail; that was hard as well, and it affected our marriage of 40 years."

They finally decided this was not a life style they wanted or enjoyed. John missed contracting and designing homes, and Rayna missed her studio and painting as well as community work.

It took several months to wind down after they sold the shop. She stopped taking Prozac, signed up for a sculpture class, and turned their dining room into a sculpture studio. It was around that time that she met yoga instructor Naomi Rose and went to her first yoga class.

Naomi recalls her initial impressions of Rayna: "When Rayna first came to my class, she didn't seem very comfortable in her body. She had issues with her back and not much flexibility."

Rayna remembers what she needed at that point in her life. "I know my purpose is to express joy through my art and life. I feel I have a new life, and a new chapter to write in the book of my life—thanks to my yoga classes that keep me balanced and thriving!”

Naomi sees very positive changes in her student as well. “She's been with me for over a year now, coming regularly to two classes a week and also attending some of my yoga workshops. What I notice now is a grace in her body and movements she didn't have before. Her flexibility and strength have increased. She has fewer back aches. Also, she seems to have released some emotional baggage so that she's come to a stronger center in herself. She reports being happier now with what she's learning from me and from yoga.”

Rayna agrees, and adds, “I find I want to send a message in my work now; before it was just using great colors, shapes, or abstract flowers and feelings with a lot of movement. My work is more spiritual now, with a message I want to share: a message of healing, uplifting, thought-provoking, that I hope, inspires well-being.”

She continues, “With my paintings my message is to bring a smile, a ‘wow’ and a sense of beauty, harmony, joy, and peace. I tend to use the *chakra* (the seven centers of spiritual power in the human body) colors which bring a sense of balance and nature as well.

“I have a different message with my sculpture. I hope that my sculptures are a reminder of the beauty and grace of our own unique bodies. Sculptures also provoke questions for me and I hope for the people who view them: Do we take the time to honor ourselves and our bodies? And do we appreciate how yoga brings out the gift of the mind-spirit connection when we quiet ourselves into these graceful poses?"

Reflecting further, Rayna says, "Yoga really changed me. It helped me open my heart and mind and expand as a person. I like the calming effects of the loud nasal breathing that sounds like the ocean waves crashing on the shore—*ujjayi* breath.

"I am instantly transported to a deserted beach, and hearing the power and endless crashing of the waves and water, and my mind opens up to the vastness and endless beauty and strength of the ocean. It relaxes me. I forget all the trivia in my life and the world. It brings me back to myself and my body and slows me down with peace. I am digging deeper now. I'm learning, growing and discovering more about myself every day."

Rayna also learned a lot about herself in the aftermath of her mother and older sister's deaths. Yoga helped her accept these changes and losses. She explains, "Death, end of life challenges, life review, memories, legacies, fears, and overcoming the unknown in a foreign environment—all came to a head for me last November."

The phone call came from a friend in Nairobi that her older sister Jan had fallen backwards down a staircase and cracked her skull on the tile floor at the bottom. She was not found for 12 hours. Jan had been the caregiver of their frail mother for 15 years, who had died the previous July at age 90.

When Rayna's younger sister Kathy and she learned that Jan had been in a coma for a week, they flew to Nairobi, Kenya, as soon as they could but sadly learned in transit that Jan had died. Rayna and Kathy began to liquidate what they could of the 13-room house and found important paperwork to help them understand their mother's and sister's lives and finances. Many friends came to call with support and advice. They learned that both their mother and sister were very involved in many charity groups.

For three weeks, Kathy and Rayna spent ten-hour days going through the contents of the huge estate. "We made decisions left and right, all the while praying for help and guidance and hoping we could do it correctly and with honor," Rayna told me. "Friends came and took away mementos, the staff took bags of clothing, towels and food, and we donated a lot to charitable organizations they were involved with."

As a result, Kathy and Rayna became closer in ways they never expected. Each evening they'd sit down with a glass of wine and go through old photo albums and review the day's decisions. After three weeks, when their work was finished, they flew back to the United States, feeling especially grateful. "Kathy and I learned so many lessons about our own strengths and weaknesses as sisters, as a team, and individually," Rayna said. "We also realized the need for support of family and friends, and the importance of faith, prayer and a positive spirit.

"When I returned home," Rayna remembers, "I felt such love, support and comfort that I was not alone and that I had my own family waiting for me: my sons, daughters-in-law and grandsons."

The only objects Rayna wanted from her mother's vast collection of art and artifacts were four beautifully carved statues of Buddha, which she was able to pack in her suitcases. She told me, "Having these statues in my Arizona home—so far from Nairobi and from Tibet—brings me such peace. And going to yoga class twice a week reinforces that serenity. Looking at the statues reminds me to be strong and remember that I can do more and be more than I ever thought possible. Every day, I feel gratitude and love."

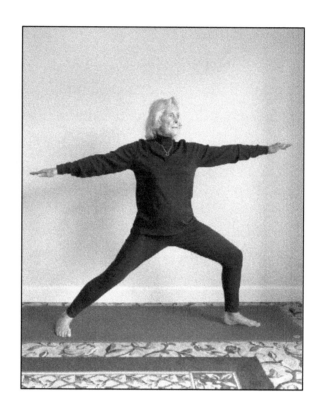

"*Meditation is my way of praying and listening. The answers to our biggest problems come to us in our silence.*"

--Susan Little

Susan Little, 85: Finding Strength

"I have been practicing yoga and meditation for so long that my body and spirit cannot imagine any other way to start the day," Susan Little told me. "My practice has been a source of strength and comfort from the very first class I ever attended 40 years ago until today when I'm grieving for the love of my life."

Susan and I are talking in my home study in Santa Fe. She has flown in from Charlottesville, Virginia to spend time with her son Tias Little (who will also be mentioned in Chapter 9) and his family. Still grieving for her husband of 60 years who died a few months earlier, she welcomed the opportunity to be with close family members in the high desert.

In 1977 and 1978, she and her husband and their three sons lived in London for her husband's sabbatical year. Once the boys were settled into school and her husband off to the library to do research, she had time on her hands. A neighbor suggested that she try a yoga class at a studio down the block, in St John's Wood. She decided to check it out, even though she knew nothing about yoga.

"It took just one class for me to fall in love with the practice. I loved the challenge of exercising in new ways in which I discovered a special kind of peace and rest at the end of a practice," she explains. "Even though I was very athletic, having played a lot of tennis, the yoga practice challenged my body in ways that I knew immediately were going to make me stronger and that the end of the practice would give me a sense of calm and peace."

She studied (and still studies) in the tradition of B.K.S. Iyengar. Her first instructor was Silva Mehta, one of Iyengar's senior teachers. In time, Mehta would publish the book, *Yoga: The Iyengar Way,* and become one of the leading teachers around the world. Susan would use Mehta's book at her daily practice over the years.

When the family returned to the small community of Williamstown, Massachusetts, where her husband was a professor of religion and philosophy at Williams College, she could not find a yoga class or anyone interested in yoga. The challenge became to create her own practice. She got up at 6 a.m. to do an hour of yoga before the boys awoke for school and she began her chores of the day. Thus began Susan's secret of practicing yoga by herself, which she still adheres to at age 85. For 30-plus years she never told anyone this story of her yogic journey, because even today there is a lot of skepticism around yoga practice among her peers. She remains silent on the subject.

Susan often wondered where this deep interest came from, whether there was a seed sown in her past. Reflecting on her parents, she remembered that they were always searching for something to satisfy themselves. However, they never supported or appreciated the influence yoga had on their daughter nor how deeply she was studying and practicing what she was learning with these experiences, so she never shared her newly discovered pathway, even with her family.

The few classes in her area were taught by teachers whom she felt did not have much experience and could not in any way compare to the rigor and precision of the training she had received in London. Instead, she used B..KS. Iyengar's book, *Light on Yoga,* as her guide.

Although her daily practice has been vital to her wellbeing over all these years, she still rarely discusses her love of yoga with even her closest friends. She tried to explain to them when she returned from England that she had discovered a wonderful program for the body and mind, but no one was interested. In fact, even today when yoga is so mainstream, there are many people who think yoga is strange.

"I've never gotten over the negative reactions I first received when I tried to talk about yoga," she explains. "Even here (at her retirement community) where there are yoga classes designed for the older generation, many who have never done yoga, I generally don't talk about my involvement in the practice. Interesting, however, that no one, with one exception, has ever asked me about my involvement with yoga. That tells me to keep quiet!"

Yet, now she is ready to "come out" as a yogini by participating in this book. She explains, "There is a kind of freedom that I have seldom experienced in sharing the journey of my yoga practice and what it has meant to me over the years. Actually, I think it's good for me to open this window to understanding what it was like to be so at peace with my yoga practice at a time when hardly anyone was doing yoga or knew anything about it. My friends thought it was just something those hippies in California did! So, for someone who for years never let herself talk about her love of a yoga practice, this is truly a gift."

Acceptance by her immediate family came slowly. Then Tias, her middle son, became captivated by yoga and developed his interest into an international career. Today he runs a school for yoga in Santa Fe, has published several books on yoga, and gives workshops around the globe. Susan's two other sons also have practices of their own. In fact, Susan chose to come to Santa Fe at this particular time so she could participate in Tias's workshop on "The Art of Self Practice," a course designed to help people practice yoga on their own at home. As time went on, her husband and sons could see how helpful her practice was to her and their support grew.

In the 1980s, Susan was active in the women's movement and helped bring coeducation to the campus of Amherst College, where she worked as dean of the senior class and director of the career counseling office. In addition, she often accompanied her husband to social events at Williams College. She experienced a lot of resistance from the old guard when she initially was trying to get an administrative position at Williams. "Over my dead body," proclaimed one of the professors to Susan, "will we hire a faculty wife."

For Susan, it was an exciting time to be young and a woman. Her early morning practice gave her the strength and courage to stand up to those who resisted going coed. At the end of an hour-long practice, her muscles would loosen up and so would her thoughts. "I was learning how to meditate and be quiet. I was trying to figure out how to have a life of my own," she says. "I was finding out what happens when we can be as quiet as possible and recognize and honor what comes into our mind. At times we wonder, why am I thinking that? My experience is that at some point, not even that day, but at some point, the answer comes."

She goes on, "I never let the negativity come into my heart. I got my strength from yoga. I stayed absolutely strong, and my kids saw that. They never saw me break down. They saw my strength and the contribution I was making as a 'rebellious faculty wife,'" she said, ruefully.

In the mid-80's, she attended a weekend workshop in Boston given by Mr. Iyengar himself. This experience took her practice to another level and gave her an even deeper understanding of the healing aspects of yoga. "My own experience, however, had already given me a view into some of this knowledge which would soon be put into action. Unbeknownst to me, I had a weak disc in my lower spine that slipped perhaps due to all the new exercise it was receiving," she says.

"I didn't realize what was causing the pain in my back until one day I was in the midst of a tennis game and when I ran to hit a backhand, the disc ruptured and off I went to the hospital. This detour did not diminish my determination to use my practice to help in the healing process, but it meant working through considerable pain. This experience did confirm for me the possibilities of how yoga can help heal the body—for, in fact, it did."

To gain a deeper understanding of her meditation practice, she began a training course in Mindfulness Meditation with Jon Kabat-Zinn, who is known internationally for his teachings. Susan also taught both meditation and yoga for a few years, but it is her private practice that has always been and continues to be her lifeline. When she retired in 1998, she lengthened her practice to two hours a day.

Susan always knew that her practice gave her physical and emotional strength, but that became more obvious after her husband died in March 2018. "It's my go-to place when I need to be quiet," she told me. "The suffering I experienced over the death of my husband was like nothing I had ever gone through. I knew what sadness was, but I had never experienced deep grieving.

"Every morning since he died I take my grief to the mat. I come with tears in my eyes and a broken heart. But I don't feel so lonely there. Solace is hard to find, but it was on my meditation blanket and my yoga mat that I gathered the strength and courage to begin my life alone."

She continues, "My practice is a big support. By the time I finish, through the tears, I feel strong, I feel quiet. I have something to hold on to. My life will change and I have to be open to whatever comes. I'm at the point now where I have to be very quiet and pay attention to messages coming to me, whether from the outside or internally.

"I know it's important for me to reach out to friends, to visit family and find a project to do—it's all part of the healing process. As hard as it was to work through my grieving, it was my yoga practice that provided me with both emotional and physical strength to go on; that continues to be so today, four months after his death. Yet there are still days when I feel the effects of my broken heart, days when I'm relieved that I can turn to the only healing avenues I have—my yoga and meditation practices."

Susan believes that her practice has kept her physically healthy all these years. "In truth, I haven't been sick with a cold, flu or any other illness in well over 20 years," she told me.

Besides supporting her physically, her practice has given her answers, directions and understanding. She explains her process: "I begin my practice with a half hour of meditation. I find that it takes concentrating on the breath to quiet my mind. Then, I often send loving, healing thoughts to those I know are in need, and/or ask for guidance on some of my own concerns. I simply pay attention to the thoughts that come to me, which are often directions on what I need to do, like call someone, write a letter, make plans with a friend or spend quiet time alone. I have learned over the years to pay attention to these thoughts that arise and I often write them down at the end of the practice as a reminder. Then I move into my *asana* practice, which usually lasts an hour and a half."

Since yoga has been and continues to be so important to Susan, I wondered what was the biggest lesson she learned from yoga. She replies without hesitation: "Over the years, yoga has given me such an appreciation for the strength of our bodies, the need to care for our bodies, and gratitude for what they can do. Meditation and yoga together have given me strength and health and ability to do a lot of things that require a strong body. Meditation is quiet time when we reflect on important aspects of our lives and what's happening in the world. Maybe you call it prayer."

She pauses, immersed in her own thoughts, and then continues, "Meditation is my way of praying and listening. The answers to our biggest problems come to us in our silence."

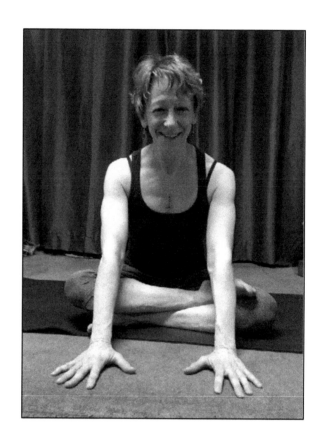

"Following the flow, the clues, the energy, that led me to teaching yoga was a practice of yoga in itself."

--Naomi Rose

Naomi C. Rose, 63: Being Present

Naomi C. Rose began doing yoga at age 13 when her school offered it as a physical education elective. From that first class, she loved learning about the body-mind-heart connection and often used the poses and breath work outside of class to help her cope with the emotional turmoil of adolescence. She continued attending yoga classes though college but when she married, started a family and pursued a career, her practice drifted away.

Ten years ago, at age 50, she told me, "Yoga called to me again. In this time of hormonal and life changes, I needed the calming, stretching, and breathing of yoga to stay healthy, flexible, and balanced. Practicing yoga kept my energy open and flowing and helped me nourish the vitality that might otherwise wane with age."

Now, ten years later at age 63 yoga has called to her again but in a different way: to teach. "I never considered teaching any kind of fitness class until my Pilates teachers kept saying I would make a great Pilates teacher. I still felt resistance to the idea, but I started getting guidance in prayer to get trained to teach Pilates. I finally relented. It was a huge step for me to teach a class as I've never been very comfortable in front of people.

"When I started teaching Pilates, I added in a little yoga. Then my students asked me if I'd teach a full yoga class. I taught one and then by students' request again, I added a second class. I've been teaching yoga for over three years now and students are loving it. So am I. I haven't yet taken any official yoga teacher training; I do continue to learn from classes I take and to study on my own. Because I'm a certified Pilates instructor, I'm legally covered to teach yoga. I may get a yoga certification someday as I'd love to keep learning how to be the best teacher I can be. But I'll wait until my guidance is clear to do that."

At first Naomi taught her yoga classes to older women who wanted help with flexibility and general health, then more students came, men and women of all ages. So, she began offering different levels for the poses, showing beginning levels and intermediate options. Her class also evolved to offering a variety of yogic styles. Titled Gentle Yoga and Kundalini, the first half of class focuses on Hatha Yoga and flow. In last half hour, the focus is on Kundalini Yoga. According to Naomi, this is a potent style of yoga for healing on all levels, for waking up to one's true nature, and for becoming more present in our lives.

"I'm surprised at the big response to my classes. More and more people have come. People are really benefiting. Some students report life-changing experiences. Something happens in these classes: Part of it is the yoga and part of it is the community feeling of the classes. Things happen in a group," she explains.

"At first I sometimes felt like I didn't know what or who was guiding these classes. Things came out of me that I didn't know I knew. Wow, I'd think afterwards, that was a good class. Who was teaching it? I was working with a shaman at the time, and she helped me learn to own the soul wisdom coming through me. She also taught me how to open up to the Divine energy vibrating through my body, especially my heart, and let it flow into the room. And so along with the students, teaching yoga has been life-changing for me too. Best of all, I get to see students benefiting from all I'm learning as a teacher."

Naomi was teaching her yoga classes at a church, but she was outgrowing the space. The owners of a local yoga studio were so impressed with the numbers she was drawing and the peaceful atmosphere of her classes that they invited her to teach there.

"Teaching at the yoga studio was another stretch for me. I wasn't under the radar anymore! And as scary as that was, it was also very good. It's a very sacred space, and my teaching has leaped forward since taking my classes there. I'm more confident now. I feel very at ease because the group is great and I'm so appreciated. Before each class, I pray for presence, to have my personality step aside. Then I allow my higher wisdom, my intuitive self, to guide the class," she explains. "Following the flow, the clues, the energy, that led me to teaching yoga was a practice of yoga in itself." The clues and energy have now led her to teaching yoga workshops, yoga hikes, and other healing offerings.

Teaching has also changed her own relationship to yoga. She practices almost every day, knowing that it's a top priority for her own self-care, and that the consequences of not practicing are too great. When she hasn't practiced for a while, she can easily feel out of balance with life. "But my personal practice is more than that," she stresses. "It has become more about other people and less about me. Even when I practice at home, it's in service to my students. Teaching has expanded my compassion and deepened my practice to yoga. All the things I say to my students are teachings for me too."

Learning how to be truly present as a yoga teacher has spilled over onto the rest of her life as well. When Naomi is not teaching yoga, she is an author and illustrator of children's books as well as a book designer and book coach. In 1994, after a powerful nighttime dream, she became drawn to Tibetan culture and wisdom. The Tibetan ways of peace and their unique culture became dear to her and soon she began work on her first children's book, *Tibetan Tales for Little Buddhas*, an enchanting book that won numerous awards and earned a foreword by the Dalai Lama. She followed her first book with a number of other

Tibetan-themed children's books. She's now devoted over twenty years to writing, painting, and teaching about Tibet and its mystical wisdom.

I met Naomi over ten years ago when she was a yoga student of mine in Santa Fe. At that time, I was impressed with her focus and dedication to her creative work at a stage of life when most people are slowing down. In 2009 she moved to Sedona. Santa Fe never felt like home to her though while living there she was happy enough. She and her husband used to visit Sedona for weekend getaways and then decided to move there permanently. Sedona feels like home.

When Naomi does a public book reading or when she works in her studio, she tries to cultivate that sense of presence she has learned from yoga. "My writing and art come from the same place as yoga—from my deepest desire to be of benefit to all beings and to all of nature. To that end, I try to follow the spiritual call in my life. And indeed, yoga has helped increase my ability to hear and listen to the call (the higher/inner guidance).

"When the call is to write or paint, I know it will somehow be of benefit. I listen to the call and let that lead the way in the creative endeavor as much as possible. When the call came to teach yoga, I responded, although I had no idea it was going to have such a profound impact on my life and on many who come to the classes. Each class I teach, I also listen to the call and let that lead the way. So often I will come with a class plan and then find myself shifting it in the moment to respond to the call at the time."

When she's truly present, she says, "The art comes easier. I'm not struggling as much when I stay present. Whatever I do, if I stay present, things run smoother."

How does she cultivate that sense of presence when she does art and writing? "I use the breath to take me deeper into loving awareness of my body, heart, and mind. *Ujjayi* breath is key for me. The sound of the ocean waves calms my mind and reminds me of something greater than the outer world—the universal energy beyond it all. And when I remember to do the breath (I often forget, but less so as time goes on), I connect to a higher wisdom/intuition, and the art and writing flow in fun and surprising ways."

The capacity to be present has also infused her ability to stand in front of an audience for a book talk or book-related event. In the past, as an introvert, she dreaded these experiences. Now, thanks to her teaching, she has a different experience. "Teaching yoga taught me that the best way to teach is to be as present as possible, as authentic as possible. So now I remember to do that at a book talk or event. I remember to breathe, to simply be. Of course, I forget too and then I'm caught up in the performance of it. But now when I catch myself being out of presence, I return to the breath."

Yogic tools are also helpful at other times, such as when she feels stressed. The minute that happens, she starts taking deeper breaths. She doesn't catch it every time, but because of the flow of yoga, she knows that this too shall pass; and this attitude keeps her from taking things quite so seriously. She knows that whatever is presenting itself at the moment is usually not a total truth. She elaborates, "I believe that nothing is being done *to* me. It's always being done *for* me (even if I can't see how at the time). This keeps me out of victim mode. I trust life and don't resist it as much. And yet, there are times when stress gets the better of me. When that happens, my first instinct is to tense my body and breathe shallowly. But once I realize what's going on, I'm able to shift to the *ujjayi* breath and that starts to calm me."

Naomi reflects on the other ways she has evolved in the last ten years. "I feel that I've come to an amazing amount of peace. Life isn't easy every day but I have more peace around it. I feel healthier in body, mind and spirit and more surrendered to what life presents. I'm more fit now than when I was younger and I attribute that to yoga. Bringing the breath to my daily life affects my health. I'm in the best physical shape of my life. I'm much less driven externally. I'm not forcing anything anymore, especially with my body. After seeing how practicing presence and following guidance led me to the joy of teaching yoga, I'm much more committed to living a present, guided life. And this brings me great peace."

Naomi pauses and reflects on the fact that she's not getting any younger. She says, "Overall, I like getting older. I feel more solid in who I am. I'm living more of an authentic life, less concerned about what others think. I'm not willing to waste my precious energy on anything that isn't true for me. I have a voice in the world now and I feel I'm of benefit to others. I'm grateful to have good health, but even so there are body and joint aches and other situations that are frustrating. And I need to pay much more attention to balance of activity and rest. I hadn't allowed much rest in my younger days. Now it's essential.

"Actually, I think there are many gifts in the aging process. It challenges me to listen to my body (as the consequences if I don't are much more immediate), to release the identity with my body and appearance, and identify more with my spirit, with my soul. The beauty that comes from aging seems to me must come from the beauty of my soul now. And facing the last chapter and end of life gives me more motivation to prepare my soul for its final work and transition."

I wonder in what ways yoga philosophy or her yoga practice or a yoga teacher informed or influenced her thoughts and feelings on aging?

"My yoga experience as well as other spiritual practices helps me release the hold on identifying myself with my body and mind," she says. "I've had many experiences of being more than my body and mind, more than my life situation. This helps me not fear death or the end of this life."

She continues, "This motivates me to prepare myself for these profound experiences. Also, I feel grateful for the opportunity to be a yoga and spiritual teacher. When the end of my days comes, I believe I will feel fulfilled that I have made contributions to others and to our world. Yoga has brought me great awareness and some skill with my breath. As in childbirth, I believe breath will be important at end of life. And even now if I find myself fearful or frustrated about aging, I can return to the presence of my breath. Yoga practice has also kept my body supple and life force energy flowing in my body, mind, and spirit. So in many ways I still feel quite young. "

Naomi takes a moment or two to pause and then adds, "Looking back, I realize that even when I was not actively practicing yoga, the early training of body-mind-heart connection continued to influence my cultivation of a balanced, aware and compassionate life. I knew then—and it's reaffirmed for me today—that yoga would be a lifelong practice. It's a way of life for me. I can't imagine life without it. The benefits are truly timeless!"

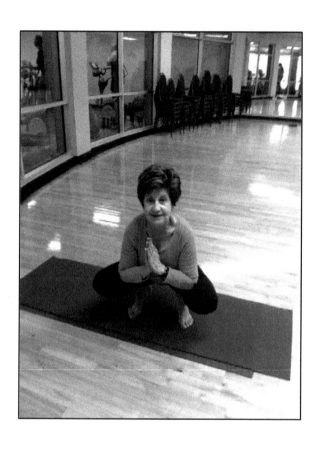

"We need to love each person that we encounter every day."

--Jean Backlund

Jean Backlund, 83: Becoming Confident

Jean Backlund had a wonderful family life for 39 years. She and her husband Phil had four daughters within six years. They were involved in church and community activities and had a busy social life with a lot of friends, including a special priest who was very supportive of their family.

Jean stayed at home to raise the girls for 17 years and then went back to work as a special education teacher when they were grown. During those child-rearing years, they moved four times due to transfers for Phil's job as a chemical engineer. For the last 37 years, Jean has lived in Bloomfield Hills, Michigan.

Jean's daughter CJ, who lives in Santa Fe, introduced me to her mother. CJ was a student of mine several years ago and remained on my mailing list. When I sent out an email looking for older women to interview, she suggested her mother contact me.

During the years that Jean was home with her children, she was very involved with their activities. She was a Girl Scout troop leader for six years, which included weekend campouts, along with the weekly meetings and special award ceremonies. Jean also volunteered at her children's schools in several capacities and at the Emergency Room of the local hospital.

Volunteer work was always important to her, starting in college where she studied to be a teacher. There was a request for tutors for children who needed extra help with their reading and math skills. As she helped these children with their academic skills, she soon saw an improvement in their confidence and in their relationships. Since then, she has volunteered in many different situations. When she was widowed, volunteering helped her focus on other people's needs, rather than dwelling on her loss.

As she reflects on those early years, she admits that she was somewhat quiet and introverted. She realizes it was her husband's encouragement that led her to pursue volunteer endeavors. "Phil was always engaged in committees and organizations. He was the one who took the initiative for family vacations and other gatherings. I was kind of there with him but I didn't take the initiative on anything. He always said 'yes' when asked to do something. I was always hesitant, due to my lack of confidence."

But that has changed, she says, when she started taking yoga classes. "I now have learned to also say 'yes,' since I feel so much better about my self-esteem from doing yoga."

When the children went off to college, she and Phil were able to pursue some time to travel and became more involved with their friends. They were looking forward to more "couple time" when he became ill unexpectedly.

Phil practiced good health habits and exercised on a regular basis, so they assumed he'd have a long life. He had no symptoms until one day on a business trip he had a problem retrieving words and complained that his leg felt "heavy." When he returned home, he went to see his doctor, who ordered a CT scan. They discovered that Phil had a Stage 4 brain tumor.

"That was such a shock to both of us," she told me. "Those six months that he was ill were difficult, although I did try and remain positive and upbeat, as did Phil until the cancer progressed to the point that he was both physically and mentally unable to function. I was with him every day in the hospital, at home and then at a rehab facility. I took a leave from my teaching job as a special education teacher."

Jean took his death very hard. She felt like her world had collapsed and didn't know where or how to begin a new life again. She went back to work but didn't do anything else. She'd come home from work, go to the cemetery and then go to bed. This was her life for a year. "I was very sad. I didn't want to do anything. I just wanted to stay in my bedroom," she said. "I don't think I was clinically depressed but I wasn't very functional."

Her two neighbors would check in on her every day. "You're not in bed, are you?" they'd ask. Finally, after a year, these friends told her that it was time to get moving and that they had signed her up for a yoga class! She was 61 years old and had never done yoga. Reluctantly, she followed them to class.

"Yoga was my salvation," Jean says. "I felt ok at the first class because I had two friends with me and I have always done some kind of exercise. The teacher was my age and she was very gentle. I did feel comfortable being there. I took the six-week series and then signed up for another series. I was starting to feel better, I was getting out and socializing. Yoga gave some structure to my week.

"After my husband passed away, at first I thought that my life would not change. I would just do what I always did. Then when I realized that I needed to let go of that life and move on, that is when yoga helped me to accept the next phase of my life. Although it is different, I realize that I can still learn to live with love and enjoy new activities."

That was 20 years ago. Today at age 81, Jean takes four yoga classes a week—her neighbors no longer do yoga. She likes beginning class with a Sun Salutation to warm up her body and make her more flexible during class. Jean also takes Pilates, aerobics and weight lifting classes. She volunteers at four different theaters as well as at the hospital and at her church. She also goes to Mass each morning. Her faith, including her relationship with a special priest, are part of her strength. "It helps me put each day in the proper perspective," she told me.

"And to remember that we need to love each person that we encounter every day."

Jean belongs to a book club where everyone is at least 20 years younger; she is also a substitute teacher. When she's subbing in first or second grade, she tells them, "I have a little secret. I do yoga." She takes five minutes out and does a little breathing and a Sun Salutation with the students. Some boys think it's sissy-ish but most of the kids participate. This way Jean gets some of her yoga breathing and poses in while teaching.

There are so many ways in which yoga has changed her life. She elaborates, "My mental clarity is a lot better. It helps me to stay focused. I have no physical problems. Is that a credit to yoga? I think yoga affects mental and physical health. A lot of people my age don't feel well. They dwell on negative stuff. I don't go there. Yoga has a lot to do with my attitude. As I said before, I was always somewhat quiet and introverted. But now I can stand up in front of a group and talk to people. I'm pursuing things that I had never done while my husband was alive. My children are very impressed with that."

After Phil passed away, she decided that she could take long distance road trips (as well as plane trips) alone to visit her children, who live in Massachusetts, Ohio, New Mexico and Michigan. This also allows her to stay in touch—beyond email and texting— with her six grandchildren, who range in age from 14 to

25. Prior to this, Phil always drove on car trips, because she didn't like to drive on the highway. She also takes road trips with her girlfriends; she never did that when Phil was alive.

Public speaking was another thing that she would not do. After Phil passed away, she joined the volunteer board of the hospital, then sat on the district board and moved up to be the president of the district board, which automatically made her a member of the state board. "These positions required that I do public speaking," she explained. "Having taken yoga, I used my relaxed breathing techniques before I spoke to a group and I was fine, much to my amazement."

Jean explains what was going on with her. "After Phil died, I had to learn to be an independent person. I had to learn to manage. I'm alone; none of my children lives close so I have to handle things on my own. Right now, I'm waiting for the TV repair man to come, and I'll deal with him.

"My mother, who died at 94 ten years ago, had little schooling. But she was a strong person. She encouraged me to do things independently. I give her a lot of credit. She'd say: 'Remember, Jean, you have to learn something new every day.' My mother learned to drive at age 61 after her husband died. I tell myself, if my mother could do this, I can too."

At this point, Jean is committed to yoga, although she admits that it would be easier to stay home and do nothing. This morning the temperature was four degrees below zero. It would have been so easy to stay in her warm house but instead she went off to class. "The minute I get in the car to go to class, I feel happy and joyful. I have to go—it's a commitment," she told me. "I love the socialization of yoga class. That's a motivation too: to be with these wonderful people. After class, I feel great. I have new energy. I'm ready to go about my business."

By practicing and studying yoga, Jean feels that she's learned so much about life. "I've learned to recognize what matters and ignore what does not. I've learned to let go of the negative and meditate on the positive. I work on being optimistic with people and situations.

"We can learn from each experience in a positive way. As a former special education teacher, I wanted my students to always feel good about who they are. When other students made fun of them or criticized them, I encouraged my students to understand that it was not about *them,* but rather about the person who was saying unkind things. I try to keep the same philosophy in my own life. Yoga helps me to stay focused on the mind/body connection. Each new day is a challenge, and doing yoga on a regular schedule helps me to accept these daily challenges.

Jean continues, explaining why aging is a wonderful teacher. "There is no 'Aging 101' course to teach us, step by step, the way to age so that we can remain healthy and happy. Only living can teach us. We are learning from the day we are born. As we age, we reflect on our earlier years, and realize that our personalities were already formed. The wonderful part of aging is accepting life's experiences and using them to build on. Learning how important the yoga philosophy has been to me is a special gift that I have been fortunate to receive.

"I have lived 81 years. I don't know how many more years I have. I hope and pray that I'll be able to attend milestones for my grandchildren. They know that I am proud of them, and if I can't attend some events, my heart will always be with them. I feel it's important for young people to know that they are loved and accepted for the unique person that they are."

Jean believes that her 20 years as an avid participant of yoga have enabled her to become a vital and energetic person in this phase of her life. She hopes that will transfer to her children and grandchildren as an example of how to live their lives, just as her mother was an important influence on Jean's ability to stay active and involved as she ages.

Her yoga teachers encourage her as well. They like to remind her that there are yoga teachers and students in their nineties, and thus make her feel like she's still young enough to continue trying new poses and modifying them to suit her comfort level. Jean comments, "I love the encouragement and motivational comments that my yoga teachers share throughout class."

Every year when another birthday arrives, she doesn't dwell on the number. Instead she feels grateful and blessed to enjoy another year. "I know that I don't have the stamina and energy that I had in my fifties, which is the ages of my four daughters, yet when I'm with them, I say 'yes' to whatever they have planned for me, and feel that same renewed energy that I feel after a yoga class. Yoga motivates me to remain active every day. My daughters encourage me to continue practicing as they see how important yoga is to keeping me healthy, both spiritually and physically. I just take one day at a time and accept each day and whatever it brings."

Recently someone asked her, "Do you do any exercise? You walk with great posture." Jean replied proudly, "Yes, I do yoga." She was surprised that someone could detect changes in her appearance from taking yoga classes.

Many of her friends have arthritis, others have hip and knee problems; some have gotten shorter. Jean observes, "I'm not different from most people my age. I just happen to do yoga. It helps me stay mentally alert. My bones are pretty good, thanks to yoga. I'm still five three. And at 81, I have more confidence than I had as a younger woman. Little did I know 20 years ago when I started yoga that it would be so important to me, especially in the later years of my life. I feel very blessed."

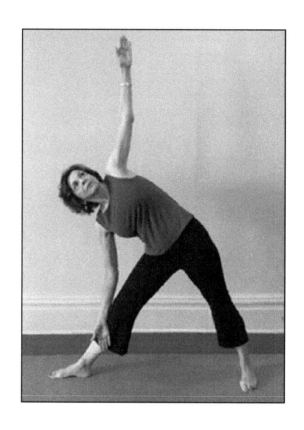

"My goal is to walk a path in which I might somehow bring some greater peace and healing into the small part of the world through which I pass."

--Elizabeth Terry

Elizabeth Terry, 70: Accepting Herself

For Elizabeth Terry, self-acceptance has been one of the most important areas in which she needed to grow, and yoga—her personal practice, her study of yoga philosophy, and her role as teacher and student—has given her the means to allow that growth to flourish.

"My whole yoga practice helped me be open to new possibilities and get past judgments. Going through menopause, I felt a sense of shame about growing older," she told me. "The physical changes of age became very visible to me. I noticed my skin began to lose its tone and even drooped a bit. Wrinkles deepened, and my hair began to thin, even though it didn't gray. And, a persistent ache in my hip required me to move my meditation to a chair."

She explored her concerns in one-on-one sessions with her teacher Fran Ubertini, who was never shy about reminding her that her body had "a shelf life" and that it would be changing. Through the understanding she developed in these sessions and with time, diligence, and talking with other women, Elizabeth was able to "get over it" and put her shame aside. In doing so, her awareness and self-acceptance grew, and she was able to move toward increasing the joy in her life.

"Bringing joy into my life diminishes the focus on how I look and shifts the emphasis to more internal things," she realized. She hoped to bring that joy into her relationship with her husband and her son and daughter, both in their 40s, who live far from her. Living in central Pennsylvania, she feels isolated from others who practice in the *Viniyoga* tradition. She and I met many years ago when she came to Santa Fe to study with my mentor/teacher, Sonia Nelson.

The sense of shame she felt about aging carried over to her vision of herself as a yoga teacher. She explains, "I had felt I needed to present myself in a certain way—thin, youthful, strong, ever flexible, master of all kinds of poses. Through examining those images that our culture presents and we internalize, I have gained a sense of freedom in letting the stereotypes go."

She continues, "Early on when I was teaching, I always had the feeling of not having enough, that there was so much more I needed to learn. And I was governed by cultural expectations. All that created stress for me. I wanted to know enough so no one would get hurt in my class, but I had a lot of challenges in the beginning. I taught at a college with 26 students in a large dance studio. That was daunting! I always wanted to be true to what I thought yoga was, but my students had their own ideas. It was really complicated: what my students' expectations were, what I thought I needed to share with them, and what I needed for myself, so I could be considered and believe myself to be a good yoga teacher."

Over time, as she worked with her teacher, Elizabeth could see she had a lot to share, particularly the teaching that has meant so much to her. She studies in the tradition of TKV Desikachar, whose father, Sri Krishnamacharya, is considered the father of modern yoga (as do I). Elizabeth had to figure out how to bring in yogic concepts that worked in the context in which she was teaching. She wanted to make the material accessible and yet convey the depth of the philosophy.

She also felt a need to put herself out there as a yoga teacher. This meant exposing her vulnerabilities. That was scary to do, but it connected her to her students. "I have to say that my teacher, Fran, was a generous model for doing this," Elizabeth believes. "I don't want to be the expert. I want to show how yoga has given me insight and made my life better. Part of that is to be self-revelatory. That was intimidating in the beginning, but when I got a positive response, that encouraged me to keep going."

One of her favorite examples of self-revelation relates to the use of *pranayama* (breath work), which is a part of every class she teaches. After she shared about how specific breathing practices helped her deal with anxiety, women began telling her how they have started to use breath work in their lives to help them deal with stress. She saw how sharing personal experiences could motivate and inspire students to use the tools of yoga to improve their lives off the mat.

She might also take a visualization or a chant and weave it through the class. At the end, she takes a moment to reflect on the practice and ask her students what their experience was.

What has Elizabeth learned from her teaching? A lot, particularly about the common struggles of women, such as doing too much and dealing with their fears. She explains, "I'm able to see these things in my life, through studying and working with a teacher, and share them with others. I've learned a lot of patience and acceptance. I'm really influenced by seeing the light in each one of us, part of what is eternal in each of us. I see that as an important connection and a way of being in the world. It's part of treating all beings with respect and recognizing our connection."

Elizabeth learned, as most teachers do, that the key to effective teaching lies in having her own committed personal practice. She explains what it means to her: "My personal practice is about me and what I need and what I want to move toward in my life. I see different ways that I made changes: how I've had courage, taken risk, sought joy. That informs my teaching: As I see more deeply those qualities and what they mean in my life, I share those qualities in class.

"In writing my blog, I might share something small in my life and how it can relate to all of us. For example, a few years ago I wrote a piece called 'The Anniversary Tree,' in which I spoke about a weeping cherry tree that had been planted on my wedding day. Thirty years later when we had to take it down because it was dying, I was angry and sad. It felt like a huge loss to me. I used the loss of the tree in my life as a concrete example of how the common experience of attachment to an object is frequently a source of *duhkha* or suffering."

Besides informing her teaching, her personal practice influences her relationships. The connection is subtle but undeniable. Elizabeth elaborates, "Because of my yoga practice, there's more space in my life. I'm open to possibilities and I can get past judgments, so there's a sense of distance. When we have more space, we can better see what we're doing and recognize when we're making judgments: Is that where I want to go? Is this how I want to be? We have the awareness and acceptance, then we can decide what we want to do. Not making judgments, I can see more possibilities."

She goes on, explaining the wide-ranging effects of yoga on her relationships. "All my relationships have gotten better since I've done yoga. I've learned to be more trusting and more open. Now I see yoga in my relationships: how we are with other people, how we choose to interact with someone else. We can deal with the obstacles by being friendly to those doing good things, and being nonjudgmental to those not doing good things. We see ourselves in our relationships: If we want to practice ethical behavior, how do we act with others? Do we have a tendency to be hurtful or manipulative? How do we practice truthfulness? Can we be content with what we have?"

She pauses and then continues. "I love these ideas—they bring home that yoga is not just about being strong or flexible; it's about so much more. How can we begin to bring our bodies home to make space for ourselves? Each of us has one small part, we're each doing our bit."

Each of us playing "one small part" reminds Elizabeth that we each have within us a light. Some say it's the essence of *prana* in all living things. She explains, "I like the idea that within each of us is a light that we call the smaller consciousness. When that light gets covered up, we fall into old habitual thinking and behavior. These mindless patterns don't serve us, hurt our relationships, and keep us in a place of emotional suffering that we know as *duhkha*. I try to remember that so I don't take things personally. I'm looking at it as awareness and acceptance. If I can accept my vulnerability, then I can accept other people's as well. That's a part of it.

"With my children, I've come to see that they're on their own journey and I respect that. That knowledge and the letting go that follows have improved our relationships. For years, I felt it was my job to make up for my past mistakes as a mother and make sure my children, even as adults, did not have to suffer as a result of the choices they made. Now, rather than worrying obsessively about 'fixing' their lives, I can accept my role as a loving support and presence."

Elizabeth was not always so accepting and wise, especially when she was younger. What was she like pre-yoga? I wondered. "I was really into a lot of trying to prove myself. I was teaching French in a private elementary and middle school and also taught in a public middle school. But I thought I needed to have a PhD. to be accepted. I had panic attacks, I was anxious, I suffered a lot. I was always looking on the outside to build the inside. I had a lot of resentment about religion and God from earlier experiences with the church. I was trying to work on my relationships with my children, I was dealing with my divorce and my own addiction. I was not with my children for a number of years, and felt I had to make up for that. So many things."

Elizabeth was 43 when she attended her first yoga class. She went after a good friend told her how much she had enjoyed it and how she'd reap the health benefits. At the time, she was searching for a natural way to deal with the anxiety and depression that had dogged her most of her life. She was so desperate to try yoga that she drove to the teacher's house, where she taught, in a snowstorm, only to find the class cancelled. The teacher encouraged her to come back.

"My experience in class was very positive. My initial connection to yoga was through a class focusing on *asana*. Since I have always been pretty flexible and reasonably strong, I felt successful in class because I could do the poses. I have never been a gym person and the atmosphere of the yoga class—low key and supportive—felt calming, reassuring, and inviting. The classes were also small, so it was easy to get to know other people. As I look back on those first yoga classes, I see that the practices touched on different aspects of my being (or *mayas*) that really engaged me."

Yoga has been a huge support for her. She hasn't had a panic attack in a long time. She has celebrated 38 years of sobriety. All her relationships have gotten better. She's more trusting and open. She's able to accept being in the present. Before, she was living in the past and trying to make up for it as well as being fearful of what the future held. Elizabeth attributes these positive changes to yoga and the courage it gave her to seek the support she needed to change.

She sums up how yoga has transformed her life: "Today I like my post-menopausal self. My practice is about what I need, not what I think I should do to meet someone's image of a yoga teacher. While *asana* is part of my practice and teaching, it takes place within the larger frame of yoga. My goal is to walk a path in which I might somehow bring some greater peace and healing into the small part of the world through which I pass. For that yoga is my guide and for that, I feel very grateful."

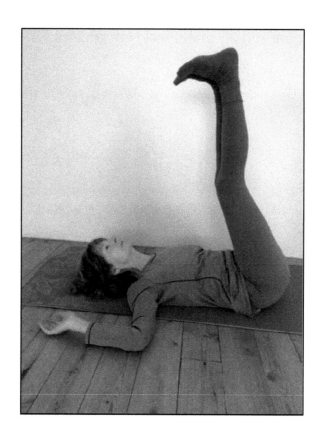

"Everything seems to fall as we age. I'm talking spiritual and mental sagging, not just physical sagging. Yoga is a counter to the forces of sagging in every sense of the word!"

--Rosemary Thompson

Rosemary Thompson, 73: Restoring a Healthy Balance

Rosemary Thompson had her first encounter with yoga in the early '90s at a wellness center in New Mexico where she worked in the human resources department of a large organization. She attended what was billed as an introductory class but it was way too hard and moved too quickly for her, as she had been recently diagnosed with fibromyalgia. She didn't return to that class, but it didn't completely turn her off to yoga, although it did take nearly 15 years before she stepped into another yoga studio.

"I was convinced that I couldn't bend over or if I did, something terrible would happen, so I'd squat down v-e-r-y carefully," she told me. "One day I was with a male friend and I dropped a nickel on the floor. I was too embarrassed to make a big production of picking up that nickel. He was standing right there. I thought I couldn't do anything so feeble in front of him, so I bent over and picked up the nickel, and nothing happened. It was a moment of total enlightenment! I realized I'd been inhibiting myself out of fear. This gave me the courage to try yoga again. That little incident made me realize, I could do it. So, when I found out about your yoga class, I thought, I can do that."

We are sitting in my living room in Santa Fe, talking. Rosemary is the student who has studied with me the longest—for over 14 years—signing up for series after series of "Yoga for Women at Midlife and Beyond." She has come to almost every session that I offer and misses class only when she is traveling. Even though she has some health issues and doesn't sleep well, she drags herself to class. She'll often tell me before class that she's going to take it easy today, but once the class starts, she is an active participant and always feels better afterwards.

She continues, explaining why yoga is important to her today. "Yoga has been essential to my health, especially since I broke my foot in 2006, which turned into a form of neuropathy. It's painful to walk and I can't walk very far. I also exercise at a gym three times a week. But yoga is one thing I can do. I'm never bored with yoga. Never.

"Yoga calms and centers me. I always feel better afterwards. If I arrive at class sleep deprived or a little depressed, I feel mentally better, physically better and the energy of the group lifts me. Sharing the intention creates a kind of energy. Seeing other people also dealing with difficulties and getting out there faithfully is encouraging. We're a community of people trying to do our best to keep going in a balanced way in difficult situations. Yoga restores balance when your world is unbalanced by chronic problems, or even temporary problems. It brings you back to a point of balance.

"The stretching and strengthening are good for me physically. All the components are there: a sense of community, a sense of spirituality, the physical balance. When I started, I couldn't begin to touch my toes and in fact, I was afraid to touch my toes for fear I'd create back pain. I'm not taking pain meds now but if I do tweak my back, I return to less pain more quickly. I've seen a tremendous amount of improvement there."

She continues, "I like doing yoga with other women my age who are like-minded. They serve as a support and an encouragement. There's no sense of competitiveness or comparing of bodies, as with some younger women. I've tried other classes that seemed competitive and I pushed myself farther and harder than I should."

Rosemary would like to have a home practice but finds it difficult to maintain. When she wakes up, she drinks a big pot of English breakfast tea and watches the sun rise. She lights a candle in front of her grandmother's statue of Xuan Yin, the Chinese goddess of compassion, and then does her spiritual reading, contemplating and enjoying the quiet. She's often in a rush to get out of the house in the morning when her energy is highest, so even though she has been up for a long time, she doesn't have time for a yoga practice.

Nonetheless, she applies the principles of yoga to her life "off the mat." She notes that they have helped her cope with stress and with her relationships. "When I remember that feeling of centeredness (I felt in class) in a situation that happens later in the day, it's easier to release it, to not get so involved. I'm not as bothered by little things or as easily triggered."

In terms of applying yoga philosophy to her relationships, she says, "I've been divorced since 1994. Since then I've gotten even closer to my sister. She's also done yoga for many years. It's a connection we enjoy and we both like to read spiritual books. She'll send me something she's been reading, like the works of Thomas Merton. We always exchange that kind of book for Christmas now.

"My daughter, who's 40, lives several states away so I don't see her very often. Every now and then I let her know I'm here. I wasn't in touch with my mother that much when I was 40. I assumed she couldn't understand my life. She was born in China, lived there until she was 18 and had a sheltered life. Then she experienced the trauma of being imprisoned by the Japanese for three and a half years during World War II. When I was a teenager, I hit the '60s like an explosion. She must have been so bewildered and upset by what I was doing.

"My own daughter probably feels the same way—that I don't 'get' what's going on with her 21st century world. I'm taking a compassionate but hands-off position. I tell her, 'I'm here for you.' I do worry about her, but I'd worry more destructively if I didn't have the yoga philosophy, going inward, all that—in combination with other philosophies and religious ideas I study. They have helped me in my relationships."

Since yoga practice and philosophy are so important to her, I wonder what changes she notices when she can't go to class, either because she's traveling or the class is on hiatus.

She explains, "Recently, I missed four classes in a row. When I got back I felt weaker, more tired and it took some time to get back. My body loses it pretty fast if I don't keep up. Another thing about yoga, if you have fear about moving your body in certain ways, gentle yoga is perfect for removing the fear of movement. But if you lay off too long, that fear comes creeping back. Over time I've learned to understand that if I haven't done it for a while, I need to get back into it slowly. The warm-ups give me confidence. Otherwise, I can paralyze myself with a fear of movement.

"On days I do yoga, I sleep better. I've unintentionally lost about 15 pounds since I've been doing yoga. Yoga makes me more body conscious in a positive way. I used to have a lot of migraines. I have no migraines now—I haven't had one in two or three years—and I attribute that in part to yoga.

"I took ballet for years so I had good posture, then all those years sitting over a desk…. My posture would suffer if I didn't do yoga. We need to remind ourselves about that: to pay attention to posture—especially today, when women are hunched over a computer. I try to make myself walk a little in good weather and remind myself to stand up straight."

I asked Rosemary what comes to mind when she thinks of the future. "There's a word that surfaces for me and that is 'vestibule.' I feel that I'm in a vestibule before a lot of aging occurs," she told me. "I don't feel I'm fully into aging the way we used to feel about it—how my mother may have felt at 72, or my grandmothers felt. They were more traditional women. They were strong but they didn't deliberately exercise or take any movement classes—except that in her 70s my mother began to walk with a neighbor."

But Rosemary sees herself in a completely different culture where walking and hiking, doing exercise like resistance training with weights or participating in sports, and yoga and Qigong make the body work more.

"Yoga has given me more strength and flexibility but also a holistic way of approaching aging involving body, mind, and soul," she says. The dimension of spirituality and self-examination in yoga, she feels, can affect one's whole life.

"Aging can be isolating. Friends die, they move away. It's important to come to grips with being alone and to enjoy and understand solitude and how it's different from loneliness. I'm more and more able to rest in solitude and find it a welcome silence," she says. "The yoga philosophy fits with that. The image of the lotus is consoling to me. It's centering. I love the way breath works with unfolding of a pose. Even with a group, it's just me doing the best I can, but that group, the core of people who come to yoga, gives me a sense of camaraderie.

"The body, mind, and spirit philosophy of yoga creates an overarching experience in which you can work to make everything about aging better. Everyone has particular health issues. Yoga helps me get through mine. If you've been ill, yoga helps you gradually get back what you've lost. It's a way to come back. It's not too much for a body."

She continues, "Yoga is good for older people because there's a lack of competition. Many women have experienced a certain amount of competition from the working world. It's such a relief to let go of competing. You've chosen to put yourself on that mat but there's no striving. Yoga class is a container, a refuge. The world throws so much at you. Yoga class is a safe place."

Rosemary notes that everyone has some fear of what will happen down the line, whether it's health issues or monetary concerns. Yoga helps, she feels, by bringing you back to the present instead of drowning in concerns about the future.

"Everything seems to fall as we age and it's worse if you're not doing yoga or something like it. I'm talking about spiritual and mental sagging, not just physical sagging. It's mostly worry that is so defeating. Worry implies projecting into the future or obsessing about the past. Yoga, on the other hand, demands that you're in the present moment and when you're in the present moment, there's only yoga.

"In that way, yoga—the breath and the postures—can replace worry with the notion of peace," she notes. "'I am peace' is my mantra. I say it once or twice and it centers me. It's an anchor back to the present. Yoga is a counter to the forces of sagging in every sense of the word!"

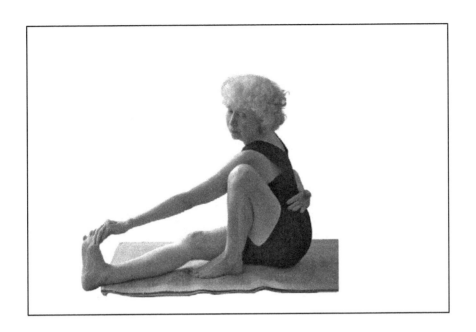

"The most important thing that defines my practice to this day is observing myself without illusions."

--Ana Franklin

Ana Franklin, 74: Weathering Grief

"My life is studying and teaching yoga," Ana told me in our first telephone interview. "Recently, I have opened a new chapter—I discovered Argentine tango! I find that yoga and Argentine tango are very compatible and I feel that they complement each other, since they both require being fully present in mind and body."

But it is yoga that has been her constant companion for 50 years. Today, it provides the maintenance she needs as she copes with the challenges of getting older. Over the years, it has been a support while grieving: it helped her navigate her life during the difficult times surrounding the deaths of her parents as well as the demise of two marriages.

Ana lives in Manhattan, Kansas, a town of about 50,000 that is home to Kansas State University, where she is a professor of yoga. She also teaches private and group classes in her home. Some people tell her that they're so glad she's there, as though she's a "special commodity." She says, "I'm the old lady who teaches yoga. That's how they see me. Everyone, both young and old, thinks their yoga teacher should be young and sexy-looking, which I'm not."

Despite the fact that she's living almost hand-to-mouth with no financial benefits from her employment and no retirement in sight, she feels very fortunate in having good health and good friends and connections both near and far, mostly thanks to yoga and tango.

Her family is on the east and west coasts and she has landed in the middle of the country, by herself. As a single person, Ana finds it helpful to use Facebook to keep up with friends and family who are scattered around the globe. She also uses it to advertise her yoga classes and to keep up to date on Argentine tango events.

I met Ana through my teacher/mentor, Sonia Nelson, when Ana came to Santa Fe to study Vedic chanting with Sonia. I thought of Ana as a good candidate for this book since I knew she'd been involved with yoga for years, but I didn't know the details of her fascinating history.

In an unlikely scenario, it was Ana's father who introduced her to yoga when she was six years old. He took up yoga in 1951 because he had an inoperable lung condition. His doctor told him he had five years to live. After doing *pranayama* (breathwork) for a month, he had a "spontaneous remission."

Ana did not do yoga at that young age but she'd see her dad doing different poses every day—it was just something he did. She emphasizes that she didn't learn yoga from her father, but a yogic spirit definitely imbued their home.

When she was in her teens, her father, who worked for the U.S. Department of State, was stationed in India. Ana and her mother accompanied him. He had an opportunity to meet Krishnamacharya, considered the "Father of Yoga," and became his student. Nancy Franklin, her mother, was invited by Krishnamacharya to take yoga classes with him, becoming a fine yoga practitioner for the rest of her life. She loved

Krishnamacharya and his son, Desikachar, and from age 54 to 94, was devoted to her yoga practice.

While in India, Ana took classes in Indian classical dance, known as *Bharatanatyam*. This interest, along with listening to the Beatles, took priority over her taking yoga classes, but she admits to feeling "a wave of admiration for this old guy." A year later, as she disembarked in New York, she felt a huge regret at leaving India and losing the opportunity to study with Krishnamacharya.

A few years later, stuck in a stressful job, she turned to yoga. She loved the physical practice and says that she finally "got" the body/mind integration. She told me, "I realized that working in this special way with movement and breath was refreshing my mind as much as it was benefitting me physically. And also, beyond my mind, there was this indwelling awareness available to me through practice."

Ana practiced on her own for several years. When she told her dad about what she was doing, he sent her the *Viniyoga* newsletter, which she "devoured." Father and daughter talked yoga a lot on the phone, but she didn't go to class much, mainly because there weren't that many classes in the '60s and '70s, even in Boston. "My own practice was revelatory," she told me. "If I'd do the simplest thing, I'd learn from it by observing myself."

As her first marriage began to fall apart, she started to spend five minutes in Child's Pose each morning and evening, then she'd lie in *Savasana* (corpse pose). She explains what happened next. "During these poses I would follow my breath and my thoughts. I began to see myself more clearly, both the good aspects and the difficult ones. Introspection became a daily thing, and I think that is the most important thing that defines my practice to this day. It's about observing myself without illusions. With *ujjayi* breathing and just these two poses and a three-mile morning walk, I was hooked. I continued a daily practice for years before being interrupted briefly when my daughter was born."

When she first began practicing on her own in the 1970s, she was overcoming mental and emotional suffering from the end of her first marriage. "I had extreme grief and found that a simple practice, a very simple practice, was huge for me. I stuck with the bare bones practice I just described for a long time. Sometimes I added some *pranayama* and meditation. Then, in the late 70s, I felt my body was strong, so I thought, why not do more challenging poses? I started doing Sun Salutations and Headstands and enjoying it—all on my own without a teacher.

"Then I got married again. My husband had no interest in yoga. We moved to West Virginia when my daughter was three. There was a community of back-to-landers that we became good friends with who wanted me to teach them yoga. They paid me even though I wasn't trained as a teacher.

"When I hit my 50th birthday, I realized that I was helping my husband run his business, but I was not contributing something of great value, which was inside of me, to the world, and that my life was already half over! 'I have to pay attention, I said to myself, I can't go another day without pursuing yoga teacher training. It's not right.' That was when I wrote a letter to Gary Kraftsow, founder of the American *Viniyoga* Institute whom my dad had influenced, and he invited me to take his teacher training in Hawaii."

In the middle of the teacher training, her marriage of 20 years was "dying a natural death." She and her daughter moved to Kansas to be near her widowed mother, who was in her 80s. "This was enormous for me. I could have gone off the deep end if I didn't have a practice," she said. "After 20 years in a relationship, I had to change *everything*.

"Moving halfway across the country with a 14-year-old, trying to fend for myself as a single mom in a strange town at age 52 puts a person under a bit of stress! I did get a low-paying job working at a local cooperative grocery, but it was a tough time. The grief of the lost marriage was more painful than anything I had felt previously, and required a strong will to practice through it despite wanting to just quit.

"It was my practice that kept me sane and alive. There's nothing that doesn't impact you on every level. It affected me physically too; I almost died of pneumonia then.

"Every morning I'd be on the mat. I'd start crying, then moaning. I didn't stop practicing. I practiced through that. When I was done, I was cleansed. I'd let the venom out and allowed the joy to bubble up and be expressed."

Ana experienced something similar when her mother died in 2010. Again, yoga helped her cope with her grief. This process has become more difficult as she's gotten older and has lost more people. But then she discovered a new hobby—tango—that, along with yoga, helped lift her out of her grief.

In truth, tango was not new to her. She grew up listening to tango and thinks she even heard it *in utero*. She sees it as connecting with her roots. Ana was born in Uruguay in 1944 and lived in both Montevideo and Buenos Aires, Argentina for the first six years of her life. It was at a time when tango was at the highpoint of its popularity, known as "The Golden Age of Tango," and it was always on the radio. Her father played classical piano, but he also learned the popular tango songs of the day and played them at home. She remembers standing on her father's feet while he would dance to the music that she found so emotional and heartrending with its syncopated rhythms.

Ana believes Argentine tango to be very similar to meditative practice and notes that meditators and yogis tend to gravitate to tango, because the feelings engendered are so similar to the feelings yoga inspires. "It's not about what you can do physically but about where your attention goes," she explains. "Before you step on the floor, you keep your eyes open and make eye contact with a partner. You don't connect through words."

She explains what happens next. "This act of being asked to dance with a glance is called *cabaceo* in Spanish. The man looks at the woman he wants to dance with and she sees and returns the glance, indicating her consent. Sometimes someone sitting in the same area may think he's looking at her. For that reason, the woman waits for the 'inviter' to approach her. You take eight to 16 beats to arrange yourself in the embrace you want. You listen to the music and your body responds to your partner's body. It's about being in the moment, every moment. You don't talk at an actual dance but you're very present. You are tuned in to your partner, the music and also to the other couples and where they are.

"Since I've done a lot of dancing, I feel more mental clarity when playing Scrabble. My mind is more acute at picking out words but also, I'm more patient and willing to consider other possibilities. That's similar to the effects of a yoga practice."

Much as she enjoys tango, it is yoga that has stolen her heart for half a century. "I'm so grateful to yoga, it's beyond what I can express. That's why I love all my teachers--Sonia, Desikachar—they plant the seeds of yoga and it keeps growing," she tells me. "I loved Desikachar so much, especially his understated way. He said, 'When you practice, things don't bother you as much.' That's exactly how I feel. When I practice, whatever happens doesn't trigger me."

She continues, "There's so much suffering in this world, I tell my college students. There is a way to do what you're doing and not be suffering from anxiety, lack of sleep, and so on. This is the path, and you have to be willing to walk the path to inner freedom and acceptance. There is a difference between constant distraction and inner peace. For me, there is no other path. Yoga has been a liberation from mental and emotional stress. It lets it go away. I think of everything as yoga."

Yoga, along with her monthly chiropractor's appointment, has also helped her face the changes that aging brings. If someone is starting yoga in her 70s, Ana advises that she should begin with a five-minute breathing practice and make sure not to get out of breath while doing *asana*. She believes that progress is less important than being present mentally and breathing well.

For herself, she says, "As long as I keep my practice going, I don't have too many complaints. I have a walking deficit right now. I feel some weakening in my legs, I've added two inches around my middle. I kept up my practice while I was sick. That was fortunate. I didn't lose all tone," she says.

"The main thing with aging is that you need more maintenance. I take warm baths in Epsom salt three to four times a week. I massage my feet and joints with coconut oil. If I dance for hours, I come home and rest. I'm always having to compensate for the things that are wearing out! For me, there was a time if I skipped a day of *asana* practice, it didn't matter. Now, I feel it, especially if I miss my *pranayama* session. I don't have the energy and my mind isn't as sharp."

Although she's only 74 and in good health, Ana has already thought about how she'd like her death to be handled. "I don't want an expensive death or a showy death. I'd like to be able to find a way out that was under my control. Some people think this is radical, but I don't. And I don't want people making a fuss. I'd like to leave quietly and be remembered as I was when I was alive. I'm here, my family isn't. It'd be good to have a plan in place because my family doesn't live nearby. It would make it simpler for them at the time but that means getting to work now."

Contemplating her own death reminds her that there are so many things she'd still like to do, but she has to watch her pennies. "I've seen much of the world and I'm very fortunate for that," she says. But if she could afford to travel, she'd visit her niece in Oxford, dear friends in Hawaii, and go on a tango vacation to Buenos Aires and Montevideo. Spending more time with her daughter, brothers and other family are always on the list.

She also has a dream for the future. "These days I dream of buying a home that I can convert into a Tango House, a place for people to stay when they're in town for a tango event. I've started a small Argentine tango group in town and I organize teachers to come to our little town. In fact, there's an Argentine tango workshop this Sunday afternoon which I'm looking forward to."

Before we end our discussion, she summarizes her life: "I've had some setbacks living in a small community and there are some judgmental aspects to it. But here I stay, and perhaps there's a reason I stay here," she concludes. "Being a dancer has always made me aware of my body and its functioning. The mechanics of moving all the joints lest they 'get rusty' has never been far from my awareness. Seeing reality takes a meditative mind. Otherwise, things can look worse (or better) than they actually are. Equanimity is the greatest gift I have received from yoga."

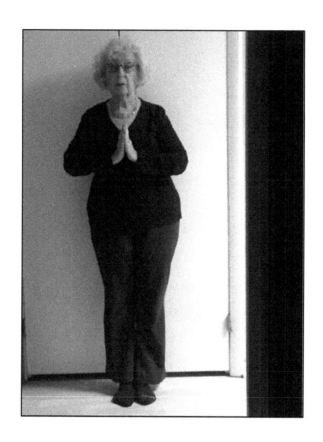

"I have a long way to go before I consider myself a peaceful person, but on this last vacation I was able to sit and watch the sunset for a long period."

--Lillian Weilerstein

Lillian Weilerstein, 83: Striving for Order

"When I was younger I made a deal with the devil never to be bored, and I paid a price for it," Lillian Weilerstein told me. "But I'm at peace with my choices now—three months from 80—and I have to give yoga credit for that peace."

Lillian started doing yoga in her 50s when she was working as a school counselor in an inner city Philadelphia school. There were many responsibilities and stresses. A yoga class at a nearby athletic facility fit into her schedule so she started going there. She decided she wanted to be more physically active even though she says that she's not coordinated and didn't enjoy other physical activities. Yet when she attended yoga class, something different happened: it felt good. This was a new feeling for her.

Lillian was not an athletic kid and wasn't good at sports, but today she feels she's one of the strongest women her age and has more energy than most of her peers. She believes that physical advantage is due to yoga.

When she first started going to class, she took three classes a week, then it narrowed down to two. Now she attends a chair yoga class once a week since the gentle yoga class she enjoyed was discontinued. She also goes to Pilates class once a week and walks. One of her first yoga teachers encouraged her to push beyond her comfort point. She thinks that's what has contributed to her strength today. "I always thought I couldn't do it. She said, 'Yes, you can.' That had a long range influence on my thinking," she believes. "I heard 'Try harder' and 'Put more effort into each position.' And I did."

And yet, she says, "I never did a handstand. You make your choices. You don't worry about what someone else is doing." This was just the approach she needed: to simply focus on *how* you're doing and *what* you're doing and not criticize or compare. When she was younger, she was more self-conscious. After she turned 80, she says, "I don't care what everyone thinks."

I interviewed Lillian several times over the phone since she lives in the Philadelphia suburbs and I'm in the southwest. A mutual friend introduced us. When she heard about my new book, she said, "You must talk to my friend Lillian." It turns out that Lillian worked at the same school as my late sister-in-law, who did educational evaluations for children with learning problems there, so we had another connection beyond yoga.

Yoga has helped Lillian cope with emotional issues as well. Her mother died when she was 50, and two years later, her father died. Her three sons had become independent. It was a time of transition. Yoga helped facilitate her moving on to another phase of her life.

"Yoga helped me deal with life changes," she told me. "I was ready for it. I had a need for something for myself as opposed to satisfying other people's needs of what I should do or be."

When she retired from her work as a counselor at age 60 and began working part-time as a nursery school counselor-supervisor, yoga smoothed the transition. She recently retired from her second career and has more time to plan her own activities now.

Lillian reflects on the changes she's observed in herself and in her relationship to yoga. "Once I hit 75 I realized that when I was younger I loved chaos, and now I love order. My training in counseling psychology made me aware of styles of learning and their impact on the individual. My learning style is mildly distracted. I am quick, which can become careless, and resourceful. As a result, I must learn how to live with my personality and I have come to like that, being quick and resourceful. I enjoyed the challenge of working with many different children, parents and teachers. I learned that problems can never be fully solved but can be worked on. It was an interesting time. I was never bored. I don't get bored and if I do, I do breathing exercises. I recognize the need to focus as part of survival in old age. Yoga teaches focus.

"My memory was always scattered though I could compensate. But I realized before I retired as a school counselor that I didn't enjoy multi-tasking any more. I wasn't as fast as I had been. Around that time, I started to do yoga. Being present is a part of yoga. I've tried to consciously incorporate it into my everyday life. I focus or try to be present in the moment: this mind and this body are important. I always believed that, even before I was involved in yoga. Yoga is a disciplined way of incorporating mind and body and helps me work toward order.

"We're all born with different temperaments. Being present with one thing is not easy for me to do. I always carry something to read. Yesterday I was on the train with nothing to read and was trying to 'be' in the place. I was quickly distracted by the view and the people. But I wasn't anxious about it. I do feel that's a temperamental thing and for me, necessary.

"To be mindful is part of yoga. During yoga I have to be aware of keeping my thoughts from moving around. It's becoming easier to do because mindfulness is a way of handling anxiety, and a goal," she told me.

For Lillian, mindfulness involves using the breathing techniques she learned in yoga class. These have been very important to her and she uses them in different forms to suit her purpose outside of class. The breath has helped her deal with simple frustrations, such as being stuck in traffic, and cope with more serious, complicated anxiety, such as during radiation following breast surgery. She's also been able to shift her chattering thoughts to more calming ones when she can't fall asleep at night.

Now, at 83, she is trying to be an orderly, disciplined person. "I have no pets but I love gardening. When the season ends, I try to make my house my pet. I take this concept of order from yoga: focusing on what needs to be done. Letting go is part of the way I think. Keeping it orderly and aesthetically pleasing is important—putting and throwing things away. Everything has its place. Moving from chaos into order."

Lillian then shifts to explain how yoga is tied to the aesthetic for her and what that means. She told me that art, music, and literature are even more important to her than yoga, but yoga itself has an aesthetic aspect for her. What she has gained from yoga has helped her to appreciate the aesthetic more. She explains:

"Whether you're looking at a painting or listening to music, if you stay with what you're involved with and have fewer distractions, you enjoy it in greater depth. I've read forever and ever with total concentration. I'm not distracted by people or pulled away by activities in the room. Yoga teaches us to be mindful and focus, so when you're looking at a painting, you're focused on that painting; you're not distracted. You're focused on only one thing. Then my enjoyment of painting or sculpture becomes part of the response to what I see and how I respond to them.

"If I had to give up reading and music, I don't know what I'd do. I couldn't live without good books to read. I also do pottery. I'm not talented but when I do pottery, I bring the mindfulness and focus of yoga to my pottery.

"My husband was very focused but he had a stroke a few years ago, and now that he has to think about focusing, he's more conscious. Things he did automatically before now he has to focus on. A friend told him, 'Now you know what normal people are like.'"

Of course, changes like this occur whether or not you practice yoga. Last summer Lillian was over-zealous gardening and experienced several months of back and leg pain. Her physical therapist suggested that yoga helped her realize sooner that she had arthritis and stenosis. Also thanks to yoga, she was able to be disciplined and conscious during the physical therapy exercises and is now back in yoga class.

Lillian recently celebrated her 83rd birthday. The way in which she celebrated it says a lot about how she feels about aging. Rather than wait for someone else to suggest a party or a special meal, she decided to take the situation into her own hands and create the birthday celebration she wanted. "What I like about aging is I give myself permission to choose what I choose to do," she says. This year her synagogue was having a big fundraising luncheon around the time of her birthday. She bought a table for her family and ten orchid center pieces at the end of the event. "I celebrated my day by giving: I gave an orchid to each family member. There was nothing I needed or wanted other than to be with the people I cared most about."

This birthday has been the catalyst for her reflecting on aging and how yogic concepts have helped her accept the changes and losses it brings. "The concept of letting go is most important in this phase of my life," she says. "I try to let go and be relaxed in *savasana*. When I'm aware I'm tensing up, I focus on the breath. That's just part of what I do. I use it to get myself started in the morning and to help me fall asleep at night."

As you would expect, quite a few of her close friends have died. At the death of each one, she experienced a period of mourning and then letting go—of expectations to visit, to talk, to commiserate. "The only compensation are the memories," she says, sadly. "The feeling of loss is always there. If there were issues, they are forgotten."

She recognizes that there is a lot of giving up and letting go that comes with aging. When she takes a walk, she's always on the lookout for a bench so she can rest. She must also be conscious of her balance so she doesn't fall. Walking on ice, as she has this winter, has been very stressful and requires constant vigilance. These are a couple of the small ways in which she has had to heighten her sense of paying attention.

Lillian shifts back to reflecting on how doing yoga for the last 25 years has enhanced her own growth as a woman. She's says she's always been mindful: "I stop and see what's around me. I probe another layer of consciousness." And of course, yoga has helped her be more mindful. She told me, "Yoga is a part of my life. It is who I am and how I became who I am. We live such a long time today, so we should live it well. I would not stop yoga no matter what. It means a lot to me."

And yet, she continues, "I have a long way to go before I consider myself a peaceful person. But on this last vacation, the sunsets were magnificent. And I was able to capture that moment. I was able to sit and watch the sun set for a long period. That's progress!"

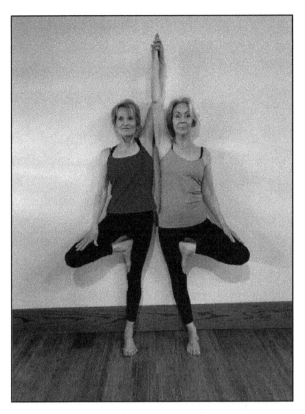

"Her heart and my heart—our hearts—are very, very old friends."

--Dottie Murphy

Dottie Murphy Morrison, 77, and Em McIntosh, 78: Deepening Friendship

There are many definitions of yoga. It is a philosophy, a way of life, and a spiritual practice. Yoga also means union: joining mind, body and spirit; connecting with the divine, or unifying two disparate things. In Dottie Murphy Morrison and Em McIntosh's case, yoga brought together two unique women and helped deepen their friendship. By sharing their passion and their practice of yoga and meditation, their friendship has reached a depth unparalleled in any of their other relationships.

Dottie and Em met when they were seven and eight years old and shared their childhood in the small west Texas town of Archer City. Dottie's parents purchased a Chevrolet dealership in December 1949 and Em's dad was hired to manage the shop and parts department. There began a friendship that lasted through their turbulent adolescence and young adulthood. They taught elementary school together in the 70s and 80s. Then Em received her master's in educational psychology and Dottie went to law school. They stayed in touch into their midlife years, and as they got older—into the present day.

Sometimes, they lived in the same town; often they didn't. Through all the decades of life's ups and downs, together they searched for a path to "true understanding and fulfillment." But nothing clicked.

Em was raised in the Methodist church and by the time she was a teenager, she had rejected religion as she knew it. Her search began in earnest at age 22 after the birth of her first son

Kirk, who experienced a severe lack of oxygen during his birth and was born brain damaged.

"Raising him was a physical, mental and emotional challenge—every single day. With the support of therapists, educators and friends, I realized that in order to find the courage, strength and understanding to successfully deal with this challenge, an inner strength would be necessary," Em told me.

"I have often said that the worst thing that ever happened to me was also the best thing that ever happened to me. My spiritual search began in my efforts to raise Kirk. I wasn't interested in learning how to live. I was trying to find what kind of person to be, and Buddhism seemed to have some of the answers."

Learning about Buddhism has been a private journey for Em. She has not participated in any organized Buddhist group on a regular basis. But through her personal study of Buddhism, she was introduced to yoga, which seemed to offer what she was looking for: the development and integration of mental, physical, spiritual and emotional aspects in the whole person.

Dottie, on the other hand, arrived at yoga from a different path. In her 50s, she lived with her mother, who had cancer, for six years. Em's mother and father lived upstairs and Dottie and her mother lived downstairs. Dottie's mother and Em's mother were also long-time friends. "It was a wonderful experience," Dottie recalls. "After doing that for a year or two, one day I said to

Em, 'We have to get ourselves out of bed. We have no daughters to take care of us. We need to look at yoga. If we take yoga, we'll be strong enough, have the right attitude and not be a burden to anyone.'"

Dottie and Em had been interested in yoga for a while, but they were never in a location or situation where yoga was available until they met teachers Tias and Surya Little in 2002 in Florida. It was definitely a case of "when the student is ready, the teacher will appear." Dottie started practicing when she was almost 60 following her mother's death—yoga helped her deal with the loss. Em began on her 61st birthday at a time when she was caring for her father following a massive stroke. Yoga helped her handle his protracted disability and eventual death.

They have followed the Littles to Florida, Texas, New Mexico, California and even to Costa Rica. There's nothing unusual about finding the right teacher and following him or her around the country or even the world. What's unusual about Dottie and Em is how yoga has cemented and enhanced *their* friendship. They continue to study with Tias and Surya to this day. I met Dottie and Em through the Littles, who also live in Santa Fe, and are close friends of my daughter and son-in-law.

As their master teacher, Tias sets the direction of their path and then, with each other as peer mentors, they take off, supporting each other during the times when a teacher is unavailable and they are practicing and studying on their own.

Dottie and Em attend the Littles' workshops and teacher trainings together and then go home and study and practice on their own. They read the *Yoga Sutra* or the *Bhagavad Gita* independently and then email back and forth, trying to understand the meaning of say, action vs. inaction or what it means to be attached to the consequences of your actions. They can have an ongoing dialogue for days. One woman realizes something and she emails the other, who writes back with her thoughts. This back-and-forth continues until they reach an understanding.

Here is an example of an email interchange between Em and Dottie on the subject of NOW:

Dottie,

One of our favorite statements by Thich Nhat Hanh is "I have arrived. I am here."

I have just thought of this as being in the present moment and that is true, but it has important consequences beyond just the present.

My reading for the day stimulated me to think about the present moment in another way. "Look upon each morning as a rebirth and we may understand that only this day exists." Of course, that it all exists NOW but what will happen in the next moment depends upon what we are doing now. Therefore, only "now" is important because "Now is the cause." The next moment is the result.

So literally with our thoughts, words and actions every moment is creating the next moment.

OMG. Constant karma!!!!

I am not sure I explained this very well. Do you understand what I am talking about?

(Source of quotes: Being Nobody, Going Nowhere *by Ayya Khema)*

Here is Dottie's reply to Em's email:

Yes now is the beginning of the path.......to choose the Result. "I am here. I make the difference. I have all that I need. I am perfectly equipped. I am the result." Yes, we are making the difference in our lives and others on the path. I love you.

While they each have other long, close friendships, this one is different because they are both on the same spiritual path studying and practicing yoga. "Yoga has affected our friendship because we're on the same journey," Em told me. "The purpose of that journey is to be the most human being we can be—mentally, physically, emotionally, and spiritually."

Em feels as though Dottie is her *avatar*. "It's almost like I'm looking at myself talking to me. It's like she's an extension of me," she says. "But I'm more introspective; she's more outward. That's good for me. We have different personalities and temperaments. We're a wonderful complement to each other."

Dottie agrees but expresses herself differently. "Since we were young girls, Em has found a quiet way to guide me to the best of all times and places. We have cried, we have laughed, and we have lifted each other up from the trying times that sometime come unexpected," she told me. "When the thunder was rolling, she could make the sun shine and the flowers grow. She always saw my heart. Her heart and my heart—our hearts—are very, very old friends."

She goes on. "When I could not find a way forward, she was the guide who led me to the point that I could look inside and see that everything I needed, I already had. Together, we have learned that it is this moment that matters—not planning the next. All I have to do is hear her voice and I know that together we can handle anything that comes our way."

One time Dottie went to a workshop in Dallas without Em. Something felt different. On the third day, she packed up and left.

She explains what happened, "It was not just about the practice. It was about Em. When she wasn't there, I came home. I missed the connection. I missed her presence and talking about the practice, seeing how it would apply to our lives, how we could live better. The key was sharing the practice. I didn't have that and I missed it."

Two years ago, Em began a home meditation and yoga practice. She doesn't attend classes except for the Littles' workshops and teacher trainings. Six days a week she arises at 5:15 a.m. and spends 15 to 20 minutes sitting and being quiet. She may read a poem or a passage from one of her favorite inspirational books. They include books about Iyengar, Taoism or Buddhism as well as poetry books by Rumi and other poets. Then she does a 45-minute *asana* practice.

Dottie's home practice is a little different from Em's. Dottie begins each morning on her meditation cushion looking west. She describes the scene: "The windows on the west side of the house allow me to see the young fillies that we are raising on the ranch. It is a beautiful view with the blue skies of North Texas and the beautiful young fillies prancing around." She spends the first 20 minutes on a meditation and then does a 30-minute *asana* practice. She takes a short rest and then gets ready for her commitments as a practicing attorney. After work, she tries to do a short restorative practice to ease the transition home from her busy work day. She also keeps a yoga mat in her office for times when she needs to refresh or restore herself at work.

Besides deepening their friendship, yoga has transformed their other relationships. Dottie has found it helpful both professionally and personally. She explains, "My husband is a successful lawyer, president of the Texas bar, a very strong man. When I listen to what he says, I just want to jump in and tell him what's wrong. But stepping back and listening has been very, very helpful. The same with my assistant who's been with me for 25 years. I've learned to say 'You're doing a terrific job on this but let's go back and look at one or two things.' Pre-yoga, I would insist, 'This is the way it should be.' Formerly, I'd want to make *me* be right and look good. Now, instead, I want *her* to look good and be right. "

For Em, the benefits of yoga are enormous. She's noticed physical changes in strength, flexibility, and weight loss; mental changes in focus and clarity, and emotional changes in being calmer and more peaceful with less anxiety and negativity. "I am a better human being, more compassionate, patient, peaceful and curious about myself, life, and others. And I feel more confident in my abilities to deal with aging."

Both Em and Dottie acknowledge that their yoga practices will change as they approach 80, but they hope to continue for as long as they can. Em jokes: "After this, there's chair yoga and then there's mental yoga. Yoga will always be a part of my life, but it will take a different form as we get older. I want to maximize what I do now because I started so late. I just keep practicing and practicing and practicing."

Dottie agrees and adds, "Learning yoga under the watchful eye and guiding touch of Tias and Surya impressed upon me the importance of discovering not only the mystery of the connection between the spirit and the physical body, but also the importance of a sense of calm, quiet and stillness. The real voyage of discovery consisted of not just seeing new landscapes, but seeing with new eyes."

Conclusion

I began this book with the belief that yoga is good for older women. I'd been teaching yoga to women who are age 50 and older for close to 20 years and I saw how much they enjoyed it. Sometimes they told me things after class, like "I couldn't sit on the floor with my legs crossed before" or "I had a problem getting up from the floor for years." Their comments always gratified me, but they were very general, and mostly about physical changes, which, of course, was heartening. But still, I wondered: How did they feel on a deeper level? What internal shifts could be attributed to their doing yoga? And in what ways had yoga transformed their lives emotionally or psychologically or spiritually?

Writing this book gave me an opportunity to sit with someone—either in person or on the phone—and truly listen and explore what their yoga practice meant to them. I expected to hear, "I'm more flexible now" or "My balance is better" and I did. But that was just the tip of the iceberg, so to speak. From each of the women, I learned of other ways that yoga impacted on their lives. Our discussions reinforced for me how this ancient practice remains so relevant and so fundamental to older women living in the 21st century world. Its existence in their lives has led to new discoveries, emotional healing, and the peace of mind needed to face the challenges of aging.

For each of these ten women, yoga opened a new path later in life. Despite their advancing years, they are still growing and learning and evolving in mind, body and spirit. This is what keeps them young and vital. This is what can keep *you* young and vital. Let these ten remarkable women inspire you, so you, too, can reap the benefits of the timeless tradition of practicing yoga.

Acknowledgments

I'm grateful to so many people who helped make this book a reality. First, I'm indebted to several people who helped me conceptualize the book at various points: when I had the original idea for the book, when I veered off track at times, and when I needed someone with whom to brainstorm. They are Margo Bachman, Gabrilla Hoeglund, Martha Jablow, and Sonia Nelson.

A number of people suggested women to interview. They didn't all end up in the book, but I did preliminary interviews with all of them to determine whether they had the depth that this book required and were articulate and expressive so their ideas were presented clearly. For recommending people to interview, I want to thank Nicolai Bachman, CJ Backlund, Elaine Coleman, Gloria Drayer, Myrna Levin, Tias Little, Sonia Nelson, and Naomi Rose.

Out of these preliminary interviews, I found the ten women whose stories appear in this book. I am most grateful to these remarkable women for sharing their yoga struggles, experiences and stories. I am repeating their names here because they deserve an extra thanks. They are Jean Backlund, Ana Franklin, Rayna Griffin, Susan Little, Em McIntosh, Dottie Murphy Morrison,

Naomi Rose, Elizabeth Terry, Rosemary Thompson, and Lillian Weilerstein.

These yoginis gave generously of their time and their thoughts. They shared their reflections and experiences through several interviews and back-and-forth emails. They each had an opportunity to read their chapter before it went to press. They checked it for accuracy and made sure they felt comfortable with everything in print.

A former yoga student of mine, Barbara Riley, turned out to be a remarkable editor. She was meticulous in going through the manuscript and "right on" in her comments and feedback. She also offered creative suggestions for ways to make the book deeper and more inclusive. Thank you, Barbara!

Lastly, as always, I want to thank my family and close friends for being there for me and for continuing to give me the encouragement, caring and love that make my creative endeavors possible.

Glossary

asana   yoga posture

avatar   a manifestation of a deity in bodily form on earth, an incarnate divine teacher

avidya   the most important *klesha*: lack of awareness/knowledge, narrow-mindedness

bhavana   intention, attitude

chakras   subtle, circular energy centers along the spinal column

duhkha   suffering, discomfort or pain

Iyengar yoga   a form of Hatha yoga that emphasizes detail, precision and alignment in the performance of postures and breath control

klesha   a negative mental state that clouds the mind causing suffering and the conditions for suffering to arise, an impediment to spiritual growth

Kundalini yoga   a school of yoga coined by Yogi Bhajan   that focuses   on   awakening   subtle energies through different practices, including *mantra*, meditation, *pranayama* and yoga postures

mantra   a vocalized sound that has specific subtle effects

mayas   layers of a person, from gross to subtle, also known as *kosha-s*

niyama   personal discipline

pranayama   breathing techniques to purify and stabilize the breath

savasana   corpse pose, rest at end of yoga class

svadhyaya   self-study, one of the *niyamas*

***ujjayi* breath**   a breathing technique in which practitioners contract the back of the throat and make an ocean sound, usually done during *asana*

Viniyoga   an approach to yoga in which the practice is adapted to fit the individuality and particular situation of each practitioner

yama   social ethics / morals

yogini   a woman who practices yoga

Related Reading

Bachman, Nicolai. *The Path of the Yoga Sutras: A Practical Guide to the Core of Yoga*. Sounds True, 2011.

Bouanchaud, Bernard. *The Essence of Yoga: Reflections on the Yoga Sutras of Patanjali*. Sri Satguru Publications, 2001.

Carroll, Melissa, editor. *Going Om: Real-Life Stories On and Off the Yoga Mat*. Viva Editions, 2014.

Dembe, Shelly. *Wrestling with Yoga: Journey of a Jewish Soul*. Health Springs Media, 2013.

Desikachar, TKV. *The Heart of Yoga*. Inner Traditions International, 1999.

Gates, Janice. *Yogini: The Power of Women in Yoga*. Mandala Publishing, 2006.

Iyengar, B.K.S. *Light on Yoga: The Bible of Modern Yoga*. Schocken Books, 1966.

Khema, Ayya. *Being Nobody, Going Nowhere*. Wisdom Publications,1987.

Lasater, Judith Hanson. *Living Your Yoga: Finding the Spiritual in Everyday Life*. Rodmel Press, 2015.

Mehta, Silva and Mira Mehta. *Yoga: The Iyengar Way*. Alfred A. Knopf, 1990.

Mitchell, Stephen. *Bhagavad Gita: A New Translation*. Harmony Books, 2000.

Page, Jeannie, editor. *The Yoga Diaries: Stories of Transformation Through Yoga*. Self-published, 2014.

Pipher, Mary. *Women Rowing North: Navigating Life's Currents and Flourishing as We Age*. Bloomsbury Publishing, 2019.

Rose, Naomi C. *Tibetan Tales for Little Buddhas*. Clear Light Publishing, 2004.

Shapiro, Patricia Gottlieb. *Heart to Heart: Deepening Women's Friendships at Midlife*. The Berkley Publishing Group, 2001.

_____. *Yoga for Women at Midlife & Beyond: A Home Companion*. Sunstone Press, 2006.

_____ . *Coming Home to Yourself: Eighteen Wise Women Reflect on Their Journeys*. Gaon Books, 2010.

_____. *The Privilege of Aging: Portraits of Twelve Jewish Women*. Gaon Books, 2013.

CPSIA information can be obtained
at www.ICGtesting.com
Printed in the USA
FSHW012251230619
59357FS

9 781644 387887